DO YOU WANT TO KNOW

—How *any* woman can attract a man and where to find the kind you want?

—What a man wants to hear on your first date together?

—The secret of giving a man a climax three times more powerful than he's ever had before?

—How to make sure a man will satisfy you every single time—boosting *his* sense of achievement and *your* pleasure?

—The sexual secret of making a man yours forever—if you decide he's the one for you?

—How to raise your own erotic self-esteem and pleasure potential step-by-step and stroke-by-stroke?

—How to make sure your very sexy lovemaking is also safe?

Now you can share the frank, sexy-hot experiences of single women just like you, plus the wisdom of one of the world's premier erotic authorities. This creative guide takes off the wraps and rips off the limits of how much fun and fulfillment is available to a single woman today.

Single, Wild, Sexy . . . and Safe

Single, Wild, Sexy...and Safe

Graham Masterton

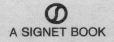
A SIGNET BOOK

SIGNET
Published by the Penguin Group
Penguin Books USA Inc., 375 Hudson Street,
New York, New York 10014, U.S.A.
Penguin Books Ltd, 27 Wrights Lane,
London W8 5TZ, England
Penguin Books Australia Ltd, Ringwood,
Victoria, Australia
Penguin Books Canada Ltd, 10 Alcorn Avenue,
Toronto, Ontario, Canada M4V 3B2
Penguin Books (N.Z.) Ltd, 182–190 Wairau Road,
Auckland 10, New Zealand

Penguin Books Ltd, Registered Offices:
Harmondsworth, Middlesex, England

First published by Signet, an imprint of Dutton Signet,
a division of Penguin Books USA Inc.

First Printing, April, 1994
10 9 8 7 6 5 4 3 2 1

ONE

Does Single Really Mean Sexier?

When it comes to sex, do single women really have more fun?

A whole lot of married women think so. When I asked over a hundred married women what they envied about their single sisters, these are just some of the comments they came up with:

- Single women can pick and choose their partners, can't they? And when they get tired of one man they can always drop him in favor of another.
- Single women can be bold, adventurous, and outrageously flirtatious—because who's to tell them that they shouldn't?
- Single women can be loyal or they can be uncommitted, whichever they choose. They can have more than one partner at once without being guilty of adultery.
- Single women can devote as much time as they want to their own fulfilment (career, sports, leisure interests) without feeling that they're being selfish with their time.
- When single women *don't* feel like sex, they don't have to feel beholden to anybody. They can curl up in front of the TV with a mug of hot chocolate

and watch whatever channel they want—unmolested.

But is today's singles scene really a sexual pleasure park for the fancy-free unattached woman—a different attraction every night, with a fireworks display to follow? Or does it exist as nothing more than a magazine writer's fantasy between the pages of *Cosmopolitan*? Does your single status *really* bring you freedom, confidence, and fulfilment—or does it bring you loneliness, uncertainty, and a lack of self-esteem?

Here's Helen, a 27-year-old hotel receptionist from St. Petersburg, Florida: "I've had three relationships that you could describe as serious. Two of the men I was involved with asked me to marry them, but both times I said no. I like my life the way it is. I've had some one-night stands—yes, I admit it. But only once have I ever done anything I really regretted, and that was when the guy tried to cite me in his divorce. I'm always very, very careful about safe sex. I mean *religious*.

"I enjoy the company of different men. I find the differences between them sexually exciting. One man might be smooth and muscular, another might be heavy and hairy—a real gorilla. And every man has his own different way of making love.

"I suppose you could say that I like the sense of control that being single gives me. I have control over my own career and I have control over my friendships and my sexual relationships. Some men don't like the idea of a woman being independent—dominant, even. But there are plenty of ways in which you can assert yourself over a man without him realizing it.

"Technique? In my experience, the single girl's best friend is oral sex. There have been quite a few occasions when I've preferred to go down on a guy rather than have intercourse. It's less risky, it's less of a physical commitment. But guys always love it. It makes them think that you're being submissive, whereas in fact you have total control over the situation . . . you even have total control over *him*.

"I know a lot of women think *yuk*! I don't want to suck a guy's cock. But in fact a guy's cock is invariably cleaner than his mouth, bacteria-wise. And once you get good at it, and you can do it slow and unhurried, it's a very sensual experience for the woman . . . maybe even more sensual than it is for the man. I love having my mouth full of hard cock; it always turns me on. I have a fantasy about having two cocks in my mouth at once, but it's never happened. Probably just as well!

"You don't have to swallow, either—and you shouldn't, if you don't know the guy's medical record. But he'll love you forever if you let him climax all over your breasts, or over your face. Men like their sex *visual*, don't you think? I guess that's why they're turned on by sex videos and strip shows.

"The future? I don't know. Occasionally I think about settling down. Whatever I sound like, I have quite a maternal streak, and I'd like to have children of my own someday. My mom keeps telling me I ought to be thinking about marriage. She says that the price of independence when you're young is loneliness when you're old. But I don't think that's necessarily so. And even if it is, it may be a price that I'm prepared to pay."

As a contrast to Helen, here's Annette, a 31-year-old resort management consultant from Denver, Colorado: "I always used to imagine that I would be married by the time I was 25 or 26. I didn't actually set out to snare a husband or anything like that, but I just took it for granted that the right man would come along and that we'd set up home together. I pictured a nice white-painted house on a leafy suburban street, a satisfying career for both of us, a nanny to take care of the children, vacations in the Caribbean, golf-club membership . . . I had it all worked out.

"The only trouble was, it didn't happen. Here I am at the age of 31, still single, still living alone in a city apartment. I've been stuck at the same level in my job for three years now, because it involves a lot of socializing, and there are so many occasions when a woman without a partner is not exactly welcome.

"I think I'm attractive, yes. I don't have any trouble with my self-confidence. In fact, I sometimes wonder if I'm *too* attractive, if that doesn't sound like vanity. I'm tall and very large-breasted and I'm very proud of my blonde hair, and whenever I walk into a business function or a cocktail party you can see the wives clinging more possessively to their husbands' arms. It makes me feel like *Jaws*, swimming into the shallow waters off Amity.

"I don't think I'm very good with blind dates and one-night stands and what you might call 'the swinging-singles scene.' For one thing, most of the men I've met in those situations have had one vital component missing—and that's the slightest idea how to treat a woman. Either they're absurdly overprotective, and they're always bringing you red roses and candies and telling you that you're the most beautiful woman in the world about a hundred times an hour, or else they live in a world of their own, and let doors swing back in your face, and spend the whole evening telling you how they dismantled their '69 Pontiac and put it back together again.

"When I was 23, I had one affair that you could genuinely call passionate. I met a man called Bradley who had come to Colorado to plan some skiing vacations for the travel company he worked for. Bradley was tall—taller than me, even when I wore my very highest heels—and very dark and good looking. I mean, really good looking. He reminded me of Cliff Robertson—do you know the type?

"We met at a travel-trade reception at the Hotel Sonnenalp in Vail. We liked each other the instant we met. I guess the atmosphere had something to do with it—the snow, the open fires. But we couldn't take our eyes off each other, and after only about ten minutes of conversation, Bradley asked me out for dinner.

"He came to my room to collect me. I was all ready . . . I even had my fur coat on. I remember he looked me up and down and said, 'You're incredible.' And that was all. The next thing I knew, we were holding each other and kissing each other as if we wanted to eat each other alive.

"He pushed me back on the bed and lifted up my dress. I was wearing black stockings with a garter belt because I hadn't been able to find any black L'eggs. He pulled aside my panties, and before I knew what was happening, he was on top of me, and his cock was thrusting into me—deep, punching thrusts like he hadn't had sex with a woman for years.

"To my surprise, I found myself thrusting back, pushing my hips up against him so that his cock went in deeper and deeper. I unbuckled his belt and dragged his pants down, so that I could grab hold of his balls while he made love to me. They were hard as golf balls, I'll never forget how hard they were.

"I climaxed first. I'd never had a climax like that before. It wasn't like a huge explosion or anything; it just passed over me, as if I was floating in a warm sea and a wave lifted me up and then lowered me down again. Then Bradley climaxed, and I was holding his balls, and I could feel every spasm. Fantastic.

"I went out to dinner with Bradley that night beautifully dressed up, but with my panties soaked and sperm sliding into my stocking tops. I could even *smell* it. I felt warm, and wanton, and *wanted*, too.

"Bradley and I spent ten days together and we never stopped making love. We made love in the morning before breakfast, we made love in the shower, we sneaked back to my room and made love after lunch. We couldn't get enough of each other.

"And between times, he was everything I could have wanted. Charming, knowledgeable, experienced—and he made me laugh, too. The night before he had to fly back to New York, I thought to myself, 'Annette, do you realize something, you have actually found the man of your dreams?' I seriously thought that he was going to ask me to marry him and come back to New York with him.

"I went to his room when he was packing. We kissed and talked, and I half-jokingly asked him if we had time to make love just one more time, before he had to go to the airport to catch his plane. It was then that I caught sight of a photograph in a pigskin frame which he had packed on top of his sweaters. A smiling blonde woman and two smiling kids.

"He saw me looking and lifted it out so that I could look at it. He was so unabashed about it that I asked him if the woman was his sister. 'Of course not,' he said. 'That's my wife.'

"I don't know how badly that experience affected me, but I guess it left me with a tendency always to be overcautious . . . never to let myself go. I knew I was still attractive. I knew I was still sexy. But for a lot of women like me, the fear of getting hurt is very, very strong. Not only that, but the fear of being *humiliated*—especially when you've been trying to be independent and self-possessed.

"I kept thinking of myself laughing and talking at that party, proud that Bradley's sperm was sliding down my thigh. That really embarrassed me. That made me feel like such a whore and such a fool.

"I'm a warm, giving person. I know that. I'm intelligent, I'm sexy. I don't even snore, at least I don't think I do. Yet I feel as if I've got this kind of curse on me, like a jar of pâté that's just past its sell-by date.

"I could make some man, somewhere, the very best of wives. I could make him happy, and myself happy, too. But it seems like the whole of our society is structured toward the young, and if you've reached my age without being married, men look at you and automatically assume that there must be something physically or psychologically wrong with you.

"Wild in bed? My God, if only I had the chance! I think I'm doomed to be alone in bed for the rest of my life!"

Annette's feeling that she had been externalized by mixed society—left out in the cold because of her age and because of her previous unhappy experiences—is very common among single women, and is one of the most difficult of obstacles to overcome.

But you will see from this book that it *can* be overcome, and that scores of single women are managing to overcome it every day.

Single women become externalized by mixed society for two principal reasons. The first is *the way that society perceives them.* The single woman can appear as a very serious threat to married women, especially if their husbands have a roving eye and/or their marriage is a little unsteady. The single woman's invitations to dinner parties and cocktail parties dwindle dramatically as the years go by and more and more of their erstwhile girlfriends get married. It's all very well Jim'n'Jane and Bill'n'Betty going off on a vacation to Yosemite together—but Jim'n'Jane and just Betty?

Even men can perceive single women as a threat. Often, they're very wary about getting involved with a woman of independent ideas, independent means—a woman with her own well-established character who knows exactly what she wants. Men lack self-confidence, too, as if you hadn't realized.

The second principal reason why single women can feel that they have become externalized is *because of their own defensiveness*. There is hardly anything that a man finds more off-putting in a woman when he is trying to establish an affectionate relationship with her than defensiveness.

Defensive women are forever making sure that they are never embarrassed and never humiliated and that they are never, ever hurt.

How many times have you heard a man say to a woman, "Do you know something, you have a fantastic figure."

And what does she say in reply? Not "Thank you" (lowers eyelashes, blushes). Oh, no. She says, "No, I haven't—my hips are far too wide."

How many times have you heard a man say to a woman, "I think you're beautiful." And what does she say in reply? Nothing more or less than "Don't be so stupid."

Here is a man saying just the kind of things she wants to hear (and probably meaning them, too). Yet her defensiveness continually puts obstacles in his way, and makes him feel frustrated and idiotic. Which— believe me—is *not* how a man likes to feel when he is making a constructive attempt to kindle a relationship with you.

The defensiveness doesn't stop there, either. I've talked to dozens of women who have pushed away men who were trying to kiss them, slapped away men who were trying to caress them, and even (in one case) emptied a pitcher of ice water down a man's back when he tried to put his arm around her.

Every single time, the woman actually *welcomed* the approach and wanted the man to continue. But, ex-plains one woman, "Something inside me just stiffened—I wanted him but I couldn't relax." Another says, "He touched my breast and I froze. I couldn't move and I couldn't speak. I was so frightened that it was going to happen all over again—the lovemaking, the falling-in-love, the walks by the seashore, the laughter—and then the rejection and all the pain of breaking up. I thought—I like it, I love it, I want him. But don't put me through all of that trauma again."

However, there are plenty of single women who have overcome their social isolation and their natural defensiveness. They have found lasting sexual happiness with a husband or a long-term lover; or else they have learned to live contentedly by themselves, taking lovers as and when they want them. It can be done, and you can do it.

Through the experiences of dozens of single women, this book will show that you can make the most of being single. Some of those experiences are wild, some of them traumatic, some of them deeply passionate.

But through other people's excitement, through other people's pleasure, through other people's trial and error, you will learn almost all you need to know to fulfil yourself sexually.

You'll learn how to find the kind of man you want and how to attract him when you've found him. You'll learn how to be witty, captivating, and *totally self-confident* about sex. You'll learn how to protect yourself against the kind of man you *don't* want to date, and how to get rid of a man of whom you're just plain tired (*without* hurting his feelings).

This book will also show you how you can lead a stimulating sex life when you're in between partners, or when you simply feel like being alone. What's more, it will show you how you can use that self-stimulation to improve your sexual self-knowledge and your lovemaking technique, so that when you *do* meet a man, you can make his ears ring.

More than anything else, it will show you that *every* unattached woman experiences tremendous highs and equally depressing lows. Sometimes you can feel as high as the sky on the Fourth of July. Other times you can feel like a week of wet Wednesdays. In this book, I hope you will discover how to make your highs even more explosive and your lows very much more tolerable.

It's your attitude toward sex that makes all the difference. It's your inner certainty.

You *are* attractive. You *are* sexy. You *can* be the kind of woman that every man wants to be with.

This is the secret that can change your sex life around, whether you have a partner already or whether you're still looking for one. Women who exude certainty in their own sexuality *always* attract men. It doesn't matter whether you weigh 98 pounds or 154 pounds. It doesn't matter if your bra size is 32A or 42DD. It doesn't matter if you're blonde or brunette, flaming scarlet or just plain mousy. You can look like an extra out of *Baywatch* or Roseanne Arnold's heavier sister.

If you're 100 percent sure inside of your own mind that you're sexually irresistible, then you will be. And that's a promise.

Now, when I wrote *How to Drive Your Woman Wild in Bed,* I was frequently asked the question: How can a man—any man—know what drives a woman wild in bed?

Just like it's fair for you to ask me now: How can a man—any man—show me how to be sexually confident in myself?

The straight answer is that only a man can tell a woman whether her sexual confidence is shining through—in the way she talks, in the way she behaves, in the way she makes love. Only a man can tell you how to be really terrific at pleasing a man in bed—in the same way that only a woman can tell a man what really turns *her* on.

I had the generous help, too, of a great many single women who were frank enough to tell me what they felt was exciting in their sex lives, and also what was lacking. They told me about the ecstasy, and they told me about the agony, too.

Here's Georgina, a 33-year-old children's nanny from Stamford, Connecticut: "I was married when I was 22 and I was divorced when I was 28. My husband Kevin was 12 years older than me, and if I can ever give any young girl one piece of good advice, that's never to marry an older man. Everything you want to experience he's already done it three times over. Everything you like is juvenile. Everything you try to say is met with the same response: 'That's all very well, but when you're older and wiser . . .' Etcetera, etcetera.

"Kevin reduced my sexual confidence to a little pile of gray ash. He was always criticizing the way I dressed. If I wore a short skirt to a party I was flaunting myself. If I wore a long skirt at home I never dressed up to please *him*. On our wedding night he forced me to go down on him, which I had never done before in my life to *anyone*, and when I almost choked he told me that I was clumsy and inexperienced and that I would never be any good in bed.

"So it went on. No beatings—he wasn't violent. But never-ending little criticisms and put-downs. Like, we went to a dinner party at his boss's house once, and when I started to talk to his boss about my views on equal employment, Kevin laughed out loud and said, 'What can a girl of your age possibly know about equal employment?' and changed the subject.

"In the end, I came home early from shopping and found him in bed with a girl who was even younger than me. God—she couldn't have been older than 17! She had been screaming and gasping so loud that neither of them had heard me coming upstairs. She was lying on top of him, face upward, naked except for her bra, and he was fucking her anally. I'd never seen that before. I'd certainly never *done* it before. I was totally horrified. Speechless. I couldn't even think about touching him, ever again.

"After we were divorced, I suddenly found myself in limbo-land. I'd moved from New York to Stamford when we married, and so most of our friends were Kevin's friends. The phone stopped ringing and I was never invited out anywhere—and some of the wives of Kevin's golfing partners even made a point of crossing the street when they saw me coming.

"I felt like a nonperson. I mean—talk about the invisible woman. And I hadn't even been the guilty party! But whenever I *did* manage to find anybody to talk to, I was always left with the feeling that I'd failed because I hadn't kept my man, and that maybe I should have turned a blind eye to a little bit of hanky-panky. After all, you know, boys will be boys.

"I was very lonely for at least six months. I tried going to the tennis club but I kept running into Kevin and one of his latest trophies, and so I stopped. I spent days sitting in the house, watching television, eating chocolate fudge cake because I was unhappy, and smoking so that I wouldn't get fat. I really began to believe that I was an ugly, awkward freak, and that my marriage had collapsed because I was too immature and because I knew nothing whatsoever about sex.

"What saved me was that one of my few remaining friends wanted to accompany her husband on a business trip to Europe—well, Paris! Who can blame her? The trouble was, her regular nanny had left her to nurse her sick father in Providence. So she asked me to take care of the kids for three weeks.

"I suddenly found myself doing something that I really enjoyed. My friend had two boys, one aged nine and the other aged six. They were funny and cute and we got along real well. Also, they helped me to get back into socializing again, because I had to take them to school, and their Little League game, and parties, and you name it. I met a whole lot of much younger women who didn't know me from before . . . and when I took the boys to the school sports day, I met Ted.

"Ted was 29, only a few months older than me. He was taking his sister's young son to the sports day for her. We sat on the bleachers and talked about nothing very much, but it was the fact that we could sit there and talk about nothing very much that made all the difference, that made me feel good. We talked about TV and rock music and why Stamford was such a bummer. All the stupid, silly inconsequential things that Kevin wouldn't talk about.

"As we left the school, Ted said that he and his twin brother and his twin brother's girlfriend were going out that Saturday night, and would I like to make it a foursome? Well, that suited me brilliantly, because my friend was back from Paris the day before.

"I went shopping and I bought myself a clinging red dress and some amazing red shoes. I had my hair highlighted and by the time Ted and his brother Michael came to pick me up on Saturday, I felt fairly amazing, to say the least. Better than I'd felt at any time since my divorce.

"It turned out that Michael's date had stood him up at the last minute, so Ted asked if I minded a threesome. Did I mind? He had to be kidding me. We went for a terrific lobster dinner, and then we went on to a nightclub and danced. When I wasn't dancing with Ted I was dancing with Michael, and you don't know how good it felt to dance like that after six years of being married to a man who thought that dancing meant shuffling around the floor to *Moon River* and squeezing your fanny when he thought that nobody was looking. Ted and Michael were both great dancers.

"They were funny, too. The way they spoke, it was almost like a comedy double-act. We drank champagne, we laughed till our sides split, and danced till we almost dropped. Ted and Michael drove me home afterward and I invited them both in for nightcaps. I played some soothing music on the hi-fi and we sat on the couch together and talked and laughed.

"I can remember how it started. I was sitting between them. I gave Ted a quick kiss and then Michael a quick kiss and I said, 'I just love you two.' Then I kissed Ted again, deeper this time, a proper kiss, and then I kissed Michael the same way.

"The next thing I knew, both of them were kissing me. Ted was kissing one cheek and Michael was kissing my ear. The feeling of having *two* men kissing me at the same time was incredible, really elating. Then Ted caressed my left breast through my dress, and Michael caressed my right breast, rolling my nipple through the thin red fabric, and I knew what was going to happen if I didn't stop it.

"So I didn't stop it. I crossed my arms and lifted my dress over my head, so that I was sitting between them wearing nothing but a red lace thong. It had been a great summer, and in spite of all that chocolate fudge cake I was very skinny and tanned. I felt *good*. Of course I felt scared, too. My heart was jumping around all over the place. But I was incredibly excited and aroused.

"Ted took off his shirt and pants, and Michael did the same. Physically, they were both very similar. They were both stocky and quite muscly, with a cross of brown hair on their chests. Michael was just a little bit heavier, that's all. Ted had a crooked white scar on his thigh. Both of them had huge rearing hard-ons. I'd never seen cocks as big and as stiff as that. They were standing in front of me and I took hold of a cock in each hand—*two*!—and slowly rubbed them. At the same time, Ted stroked my hair and Michael caressed my shoulders.

"For a moment, I was terrified that Kevin had been right about me, and that I was too inexperienced to give a man any satisfaction—let alone *two* men. But I could tell by the way that Ted and Michael were responding that they were enjoying me rubbing their cocks. I was giving them long, hard, slow strokes, and circling my thumb around the openings. The skin stretched backwards and forwards, and the heads of their cocks were deep crimson and looked as if they were about to burst.

"Both of them started to get slippery with lubricant, so I rubbed both of their cock-heads together, around and around, until they were all glistening and wet.

"It was then that Ted gently guided me down onto the rug. I lay on my back while Michael knelt over my head. I could see his balls and his cock rearing up above me, so I reached up and pulled it downwards, licking and kissing it, and sucking all the lubricant off. He didn't force me to do it—I wanted to, to please him, and because it tasted delicious.

"Both of them tugged my thong out from between the cheeks of my bottom. While Ted pulled it off over my ankles, Michael opened up my pussy with both hands. Actually it's not a 'pussy' in the summer because I always shave. I lifted my head and looked down, and I could see my bare pussy stretched wide apart by Michael, so that my clitoris stuck up, pink and exposed; and Ted kneeling between my thighs with his hard cock in his hand, ready to slide it into me.

" 'Uh-oh, condoms!' Michael warned his brother. With his stiff cock bobbing only a few inches above my face, he turned around and reached into his jeans pocket and took out a pack of Trojans. I watched as

Ted unrolled his condom over his cock, and—right above me—as Michael rolled his on, too.

"Michael caressed my breasts, massaging them around and around, while Ted leaned over me and kissed me, licking my tongue, licking my teeth, licking my lips. Then, very slowly, he slid his cock into my pussy, and I can't tell you how beautiful that felt. I could feel every inch of it sliding up inside me, hard and cool and slippery, until his pubic hair was prickling against my bare-shaved pussy, and his balls were joggling against the cheeks of my bottom.

"He slid oh-so-slowly in and out, teasing me, taunting me. All I wanted was that huge great cock right up deep inside me, but he kept dipping just the head of it in, and then taking it out again. I could hear how juicy my pussy was getting—every time he slid his cock in, it made a sound like a wet kiss.

"I seized hold of his bottom in both hands, and dug my nails into him, and forced him to push himself deeper inside me. Then I forced him again and again. I didn't care if I hurt him, I just wanted that cock so deep inside me that I could feel it in my throat.

"Ted fucked me like that for a few minutes, and then took his cock out and lay on his side on the rug, next to me. He kissed me and stroked my hair and told me how pretty I was . . . and I had Michael nuzzling my neck and telling me that he'd never met another girl like me. I was delirious!

"Michael lay down on the rug behind me. I could feel his hairy chest against my back. He lifted my thigh with his hand, and slowly slid his cock into my pussy. I closed my eyes. That was fantastic—one cock after another. But then he took it out again, all slippery with pussy juice, and I felt him pressing it against my anus.

"I suddenly thought of Kevin lying on my bed with that young girl, with his cock inside her ass, and I reached behind me and tried to push him away.

"But Ted kissed me again and said, 'Try it, you'll like it.'

"Michael pressed the head of his cock up against my anus again. Ted reached around and smeared more juice on it, and then gently probed his finger into it. I flinched and tightened, but Ted said, 'Ssh, all you have to do is push *against* it.

"I pushed against it, and Ted probed another fingertip into it. Slowly, he stretched my anus open so that his brother could push the head of his cock into it.

"To begin with, I felt a wince of pain, and I almost panicked. I thought, 'I *can't*, I simply *can't*. But then I pushed against it, the way that Ted had told me, and this whole huge cock slid into my bottom, right up to the balls, and it gave me a sensation like nothing I'd ever, ever felt before.

"Ted eased himself closer. He was kissing me all the time, tangling his fingers in my hair, telling me how exciting I was. He slid his cock into my pussy, and then I had two cocks deep inside me, both at once, pushing up and down, rubbing up against each other, jostling for space inside my stretched-open pussy and my stretched-open ass.

"I reached down and felt *four* hard hairy balls between my legs. I rolled them with my fingers, and ran my fingers around the slippery tight skin where all three of us joined together. Michael climaxed first. He clung on to me and shuddered, and I was sure that I could actually feel his condom bulging up inside my ass. That started me off—I had a tight, quivering kind of orgasm like an electric shock. Every single muscle in my body seemed to tense up.

"Then Ted came, too, and we all held on to each other for what seemed like hours, panting and kissing and gradually relaxing.

"I never dated either Ted or Michael ever again, and I don't think I'd ever consider making love to two men ever again. Not both at the same time, anyway! I thought for a while that it might have been sluttish and sinful of me to do what I did. But then I thought, I'm a free woman, I can do what I like, so long as I don't hurt anybody.

"I began to realize that Ted and Michael had given me back my sexual confidence. I *knew* that I was sexy. I knew that I could satisfy a man. In fact, I knew that I could satisfy *two* men. One guy came up to me in a singles bar not long after and said, 'I bet you're not enough woman for *me*, darling!' and I thought, 'Oh, yes I am, you and another one like you.'

"I think I learned from Ted and Michael that sex wasn't anything to be afraid of. It's for pleasure. It's for expressing affection—and, if you're lucky, it's for expressing love.

"Of course the other good thing that happened was that my friend gave me an excellent reference, and I've since had two other jobs as a nanny. It's a way of getting to meet people, a way of keeping yourself socially involved, a way of being part of a family—which, when you're divorced, is one of the things you miss the keenest.

"I have a man friend now, a real quiet, calm gentleman called Richard. I don't know whether I'll ever marry him, but I know that I please him, just the way that every woman with enough sexual confidence can please *any* man."

Before you start getting worried, taking part in a three-in-a-bed session is certainly not necessary for restoring your sexual confidence, and is very much further than most single women are normally prepared to go. For most single women, a loving and exciting encounter with one attractive man is all they need.

In fact, there is nothing to stop you from recharging the batteries of your sexual self-assurance before you manage to find anybody at all. You might be alone, but that doesn't mean for a moment that you have to be stale. This book will show you how to satisfy yourself in several highly pleasurable and very special ways, and how to prepare yourself for future sexual encounters.

If you can regain your sexual self-confidence, you can turn your whole romantic life right around—back to the days when you always had a lover and when love was something you shared in, too. Or—if you've never had a lover—this book can tell you how to find one, and what to do when you've got one.

- You can attract the kind of man you really want. You don't have to compromise!
- You can please him when you've got him—in fact, he'll never want to let you go!
- You can build a long-term relationship that never lacks for excitement.

When I suggested to dozens of single women that they really could attract, excite, and *keep* the men they fell for, about eighty percent refused to believe me. They'd gotten so locked on to the idea that they weren't attractive anymore, that they were homely and unwanted failures.

Well, this book is designed to unlock all of that defensiveness, all of that reserve, all of that feeling that "I'm still single, so nobody wants me." Somebody *does* want you. Somebody can't wait to take you into his arms and love you. He's out there, and you can find him, and you can have the kind of love life you always dreamed about. *If* you're prepared to be adventurous. *If* you're prepared to lower some of those defenses of yours.

If you're prepared to let go.

What do I mean by "let go"? Later, I'll give you a simple and effective program that is designed to build up your sexual confidence by yourself, at home, and in complete privacy. Let's put it this way: Nobody will know that you're doing it, but by the time you've finished doing it, your skill in sex will be dramatically improved . . . and, believe me, you'll enjoy it, too.

You see, first of all, you have to learn how to be comfortable with yourself. Sexually, I mean. Then you can learn how to be comfortable with men.

I'll be asking you to do things that you never considered before. Maybe you were always too shy. Maybe you thought that they were "dirty." Maybe you thought that you were compromising yourself and your moral values.

Just remember: You're always entitled to your own beliefs about sex and sexual behavior. I never want to question that. But there has never been anything etched in marble that denies you the right to the erotic pleasures of your own body. And there has never been anything etched in marble that denies you the right to companionship, affection, and love.

In fact, I'd like to have it chiseled in marble that every woman everywhere, if she wants to, is entitled to wake up in the morning next to a man she adores. And if she wants to wake up on her own, then she should always wake up with a smile on her face.

Let me put my own sexual philosophy into one sentence: If it excites you, if it brings you happiness and satisfaction, and if nobody is hurt or put at risk, either physically or emotionally—then do it. The results can be extraordinary.

But what if you've suffered some really hard knocks? What if your sexual confidence has been shaken by some very demoralizing setbacks?

We've heard about Georgina's "high" with Ted and Michael. Now let's hear from Hedda, a 28-year-old nurse from Los Angeles who had a less-than-happy experience after responding to a personal ad placed by a "SWM, 5' 11", 174, non-smoking, good-looking, self-employed, semiretired by choice, seeks younger lady who knows the power of her own femininity for long-term romance and possible family. Must enjoy driving to the beach in a pristine 450SL, Mexican food, Pinot Grigio, the sound of the surf, diversity."

"He sounded well off, self-assured, and he didn't sound like he was afraid of a woman with a personality. My love life had been at a pretty low ebb for almost a year, because I'd finished a three-year relationship with a man I really liked. In fact, if you want the truth, a man I really *loved*.

"*That* relationship had come to grief because he couldn't stand me being opinionated and political. As far as he was concerned, women were for decorative purposes only. He loved walking into a restaurant with me hanging on his arm, and he loved it when I wore short skirts and low tops and tiny bikinis. He used to say, 'Look at those guys . . . their tongues are hanging out so far you could wipe your feet on them.'

"I hated all of that, but I loved him and when you love a man, you kind of lose your sanity, don't you? Especially when you're young and inexperienced, like I was. The only thing I *couldn't* stand was his sleeping with other women. He went out with other girls about two or three times in the first year we were living to-gether. When I complained about it, he used to say that we weren't married, were we?—and that I was just as free to go out with other men. Mind you, I can just guess what his reaction would have been if I *had* gone out with another man.

"His unfaithfulness got worse and worse. I used to come home sometimes and find other girls in our bed, or the sheets rumpled up and stinking of perfume and sex and sweat. In the end, I simply packed my bags and left. He was hurt. He was amazed. He was angry. He kept saying 'What have I done? What have I done?' And I thought, what you've done is take my pride, my self-esteem, my happiness, my individuality, and a whole lot of my money, too. You've treated me like a centerfold in a sex magazine. All that's missing are the staples in my stomach.

"When I was living with him, I used to see unattached girls flirting around and having a whole lot of fun. But now that *I* was single, I was nothing but depressed. I was so depressed that after a while none of my friends used to call me anymore, because I was such a drag to be with. I went through every day with a heart like lead, feeling lonely and listless and no good to anybody.

"Then I met a woman patient in the hospital whose husband used to come visit her every single day, and bring her flowers and books and gifts and all kinds of stuff. I happened to make a remark about how happy they were, and I was really surprised when she told me that they had met through a personal ad. She said I should try looking through some of the magazines, and answer some of the ads that caught my eye. So that's what I did, and that's how I met up with Ralph.

"When he said 'good-looking' in his advertisement, he was stretching the truth a little. He wasn't 'good-looking' in the sense that Kevin Costner is good looking or Tom Cruise is good looking. He was more good looking in the sense that Jeff Goldblum is good looking. He was a *very* snappy dresser. Armani suits, the whole bit. And the Mercedes was real. I never quite found out what he did for a living. He said it was something to do with boats—but, whatever it was, he was obviously making quite a lot of money out of it.

"We dated, he took me to dinner. He said he had never expected to meet anybody so pretty through a personal ad. He said he had always wanted to settle down and have a family, but there had always been too much pressure of work, and now he found it difficult to meet the kind of woman he had always dreamed of.

"He was every inch the gentleman. He didn't try anything—not on that first date, anyway. He kissed me on the doorstep when he took me back to my apartment, but that was all. We agreed to meet again, and the next time he was much more romantic. He said he'd known me only a few hours, but already he felt that he was in the presence of a kindred soul. Something like that.

"He took me back to his apartment. It was a huge place on Santa Monica, not far from Century City. It had thick-pile rugs, paintings and sculpture everywhere. We sat in front of the open fire and shared a bottle of Dom Perignon. He played some schmaltzy music . . . not quite to my taste, I'm afraid. I prefer Z. Z. Top, but I didn't tell him. We kissed, and started getting ourselves pretty well worked up.

"He produced a beautifully wrapped box and when I opened it, there was a silky peach-colored negligée inside. He'd bought it on Rodeo Drive, and it must have cost him a fortune. I refused it at first because I didn't want to feel compromised, but in the end I accepted it because I didn't want to hurt his feelings.

"He asked me if I wanted to try it on, and I said for sure. So I went to the bedroom and undressed and brushed out my hair and sprayed myself with perfume, and I have to tell you that I looked pretty good. As a matter of fact, I must have gotten my self-confidence back in spades, because I thought I looked sexier and more attractive than anyone that Ralph could have found for himself by any other means apart from a personal ad.

"I went back to the living room and Ralph was totally knocked out. We drank more champagne, we listened to more music. He kissed me and caressed my breasts through the negligee, and I didn't resist. I wanted to feel that a man wanted me. He laid me down on the cushions in front of the fire, and I unbuttoned his shirt and stroked his chest. He had a good, firm body. He must have worked out every day. I unbuckled his belt for him, and he took off his pants.

"He kissed me and squeezed my nipples and bit at my ears. He was very passionate—a really heated Latin-style lover. He kept murmuring that I was so beautiful, that my skin was so creamy, that my breasts were so firm, that my thighs were so warm. I loved it: It turned me on. I had never had a man say anything like that to me before.

"He lifted my negligée and kissed my stomach and my thighs, and then he kissed my vagina. I had never had a man do *that*, either, and to begin with I didn't know how to react. My previous boyfriend would never have done that to me. He would have considered it demeaning to lick a woman's vagina . . . all he ever wanted was for me to suck his penis . . . and I wouldn't do that very often. I always used to wonder if it had been in another woman before he put it in my mouth.

"Anyway, Ralph was turning me on like you can't believe. He was licking and sucking my clitoris, he was wiggling the tip of his tongue into my vagina. He was giving me feelings that I'd never had before. He opened my vagina wide with his fingers and gently sucked my lips into his mouth. I had never realized that a man could make me feel this way.

"He stopped licking me, and knelt between my legs. His penis was hard, and I reached down and stroked it two or three times. He was just about to push himself inside me when I said, 'Ralph . . . condom, Ralph.'

"He froze. He said, 'I don't want to wear a condom, honey. I hate them.'

"I said, 'I can't let you make love to me without a condom.'

"He said, 'I'm not HIV positive, if that's what you're trying to suggest.'

"I said, 'I'm not trying to suggest that you're HIV

positive. I'm just protecting myself, the same way that every woman has a right to protect herself. The same way that you have a duty to protect yourself. Either of us may be HIV positive without knowing it. You may have another medical problem that you don't know about—herpes or something like that.'

"Ralph went crazy. He said, 'Look what you've done now . . . you've turned a romantic evening into a god-damned seminar on disgusting diseases!'

"But I said, 'If you'd put on a condom, the problem wouldn't have come up. You should wear a condom. It's good sexual manners, it's etiquette. Besides, I'm not on the pill. I don't have an IUD. You could make me pregnant.'

"He went double-crazy. 'I went down on you and I didn't ask you if you were HIV.'

"I said, 'You can't catch AIDS from licking a woman's vagina.'

" 'And so what if you did get pregnant? You know that I want to start a family!'

" 'Come on, now,' I told him. 'If I want to start a family, I want to start it by choice, and not by carelessness.'

"Well, he said he was sorry, and he hadn't meant to bully me. But he said he'd fallen in love with me, and wanted to marry me . . . and if I got pregnant sooner rather than later, what did it matter? I told him it mattered because I had a career. I was a fully qualified nurse, with terrific prospects in advanced health care.

"Do you know what he did? He laughed. He said, 'I wouldn't expect you to *work*, once we get married! A pretty little thing like you!'

"It was then that I knew that I'd walked straight back into the same kind of relationship that I'd had with my ex-boyfriend, all over again. As far as he was concerned, I was a toy, a plaything—no more or less desirable than his Mercedes.

"Of course, that was pretty much the end of the evening and pretty much the end of our dream relationship. I was back to being single, and back to being alone. One good thing, though: I wasn't depressed anymore, so the experience wasn't wholly wasted. I knew now that the fault in my love life wasn't me. I was sexy, warm, and willing, but not at the cost of losing my individuality or my dignity—or my life, come to that.

"I also learned to ignore any personal ad which contains even a hint of materialistic boasting. 'I have a house on the beach and a private plane.' Forget it. If a guy with a house on the beach and a private plane has to place a personal ad for female companionship, then he must be seriously deficient in some department. Best left alone, before you find out what that deficiency is.

"I also learned that I have the strength to say 'no' to a man when I want to. I should have told him that I hated his music. I should have told him that I didn't like Dom Perignon. I never wear negligées, either. They're just not my style.

"I didn't dislike him. I could have loved him, I think. But there was no way in the world that I was going to allow another man to treat me like a decorative appendage, without opinions of my own, without tastes of my own, without a life of my own."

At the time I talked to her, seven months after this experience, Georgina was still single and living alone, but she had a man friend who was "funny, sweet, and very good to me," and she was feeling much more confident, sexually whole, and "pretty much pleased with myself."

The most important message of Georgina's experience, without any doubt, is that a single woman should do whatever she can to achieve this sense of inner confidence, sexual wholeness, and self-acclaim. Single women of any age can be freer and sexier—and have a much greater chance of success with men—if they *don't* carry with them the luggage of previous romantic failures, and if they feel no sense of panic or desperation whatsoever. Your time is coming—guaranteed!

Later, we'll be looking in detail at personal ads and other ways of meeting men, like dating agencies and lunch clubs and singles lines. But however you try to find a partner, you should arrive on those dates full of sexual self-assuredness—certain of your worth, certain of your attractiveness.

You should also be certain of what it is that you want—so many single women simply don't have any idea! And you should have the confidence to say "yes" when you find it, and "no" when you *don't* find it.

These are not just words. These are real goals, which you can achieve very quickly by practical self-education and sensible self-appraisal—by facing up to some of the things in your sex life that you may not have wanted to face up to before.

Believe me, this self-education and self-appraisal isn't frightening, either. It can be challenging, yes, but most of the time it's highly enjoyable.

Do you know what a man most wants to hear on your first date together? Do you know what sexual signals you can give to a man to evoke the strongest and fastest response? Do you know what kind of clothing a man likes most when he's meeting a woman for the first time?

Do you know the secret of giving a man a climax three times more powerful than he's ever had before? Do you know how to make sure that a man will satisfy you every single time you make love, boosting *his* sense of achievement and *your* pleasure? Do you know the sexual secret of making a man yours forever—*if* you want him? (Don't try it if you *don't* want to see him again—he'll pester you forever after!

When I wrote *How to Drive Your Woman Wild in Bed* a few years ago, I was asked by television interviewers how I knew what it was that makes a woman feel aroused, excited, and sexually satisfied. After all, I'm a man, and with the best imagination in the world, I can never know what it's like to experience a female orgasm, or to be vaginally penetrated by a man's penis.

The simple answer is that over my quarter-century of sexual counseling I have asked literally hundreds of women what it is, sexually, that they enjoy the most. Women are almost always forthcoming about what they like in bed—much more forthcoming than men. I had only to ask, and then to listen. The interesting part about it was that most of what women wanted wasn't what other sex books said they wanted, or even what articles in sophisticated women's magazines said they wanted.

At that time (in mid-1970s), most sex books were written by men who had made totally unfounded assumptions about what women wanted out of a sexual relationship, without bothering to ask them. (For instance, I have a 1970s sex book that says "Women over the age of 45 generally lose most of their interest in sex." Another one asserts, "The penis should be thoroughly washed every day and coated in talcum powder"!!!) Other sex books of that period were written by women who had a strong feminist ax to grind.

I can understand the feminist ax grinding. In fact, I wouldn't mind seeing more of it today. There is a whole new generation of young women reaching sexual maturity who would benefit enormously from the kind of consciousness raising that revolutionized sexual relationships in the Sixties, Seventies, and Eighties. Some of that consciousness raising was misguided; some of it may have been hysterical. But on the whole it advanced women's status in sexual relationships to the point where every woman knows that she has a right to sexual pleasure, sexual happiness, and to enjoy herself in bed without feeling threatened or degraded.

In the same way, I've talked to dozens and dozens of single women in order to find out what sexual problems you *really* face. And I've talked to dozens of experienced people who work for dating services and contact magazines and who regularly deal with single people who are looking for love.

Just before starting this book, I had lunch with a very talented young lady who started her own millinery business from scratch. She had the prettiest face, the most beguiling smile, and she also happened to be tall and heavily built. During the course of the conversation, I described a friend of mine as fat. This young lady's response was instantly defensive. "What's wrong with being fat?" she wanted to know, in a hostile tone.

This response had two negative effects. It immediately told me that she was self-conscious about her size, and that before any man could have any kind of easy relationship with her—even a casual friendship— the problem of her size would have to be discussed at a fundamental level.

It also put me in a position where I had to defend my view of the world and the people in it before our conversation could continue. As it happens, my friend happens to know that he's fat, and doesn't mind being fat, and as far as I'm concerned and he's concerned, "fat" is an accurate and non-sizeist description. A Sumo wrestler would think my friend is a runt, but he's fat compared with most of the world's population. And do you know what? It doesn't matter. Any more than this girl's fatness mattered. I happen to like fat girls, except when they give me a hard time for calling them fat.

This is why I say be happy about yourself before you start looking for anybody new. Don't expect a new partner to solve all your sexual and emotional problems for you. They probably won't want to. They probably can't.

The most important thing to remember is that even in your lowest moments—when you feel that nobody loves you and that you're not likely *ever* to find anyone who does—you're not alone. There are always people who understand, as you will see from the firsthand personal accounts that I've collected for this book.

Compare your own experiences with those of Anna, a 26-year-old legal secretary from Boston who is pretty, bright, and sexy: "My mother brought me up to believe that we live in a brave new world of sexual equality. From the time that I reached puberty, she taught me that my sexual needs were natural and normal. She taught me to how to respect my body. She taught me how to dress well. She taught me how to talk to men. As I grew older, she discussed everything from masturbation to oral sex.

"She always used to say to me, 'You're not going to make the same mistakes that *I* made. You're going to be knowledgeable; you're going to know what you want. You're going to meet a terrific guy. You're going to get married, you're going to be happy, you're going to be satisfied.'

"And do you know what? I've never been married, I've never been happy, and most of all I've never been satisfied. My first experience of sex was in the back of an Oldsmobile with a pimply college senior who came all over my best velvet skirt. My next experience of sex was four months of living with a science lecturer who hit me.

"Then I met a publisher who was caring and kind and experienced—and married. By the time I was 23 I was feeling all burned out, as if I'd *never* meet the right man. I felt totally excluded from normal society, from normal men and women. I began to think that there was something wrong with me. Maybe I was ugly without realizing it. Maybe I came on too confident and scared men away.

"My self-esteem went down to absolute zero. Below zero, if that's possible. I began to dress drably and carry myself drably. I went through 13 months of despair.

"Then I picked up a copy of a magazine at a friend's house and read through the personal columns. You know the kind of thing. 'DWM—tall, dark, handsome, successful and kind, 5' 9", seeks beautiful professional woman who is as wonderful as me.'

"I took the magazine home with me. In fact, I'm ashamed to say that I stole it. I looked through the personals and I was totally *amazed* how many there were. I mean, even if you believe only *half* of what these people say about themselves, they still sound incredibly eligible. Wealthy, funny, attractive, non-smoking, considerate, generous, *voguish,* for God's sake.

"Out of curiosity, out of loneliness, I answered three of the advertisements and decided to meet two of the men who answered. One was insufferably vain. He spent the whole of dinner talking about himself. I thought: No wonder you're single. But afterwards, of course, I was full of remorse. Maybe I was still single for the same reason.

"On the next date, I met a man who was so unlike any man I'd ever known before that I nearly turned around and walked right out of the restaurant the second I saw him. I'm small and blonde and energetic. He was tall and dark and very, very quiet. But, do you know, once I started talking to him, I began to like him a whole lot. He was so *different*, so unusual . . . and so attractive.

"All of my life, without even realizing it, I'd been looking for a man just like my father. All of my life I'd been looking for the kind of man who would have made my mother happy. What I needed was a man whose outlook on life was completely unfamiliar—a man who was going to broaden my outlook. I found such a man through a personal ad in a magazine and I'm not ashamed to admit it.

"We had dinner two or three times, then he took me boating. The next weekend he asked me to stay for the weekend at an inn in Chatham. I said, um, yes—and that was when we started sleeping together.

"All of those things that my mother had told me about—kissing, caressing, massage, oral sex—they all came into focus. They all made sense. We had a fantastic weekend together—walking, making love, swimming, making love, yachting, making love . . .

"It's the right partner that makes all of the difference. It's the right partner that makes sex sexy. Maybe if my mother had told me that, I would have saved myself a whole lot of grief. Sexual equality doesn't mean anything unless you have a partner you want to whom you want to be equal."

I know that you're going to find something, somewhere in this book that will give you sexual confidence in yourself. A little spark of inspiration—that's all it takes.

Try some of the exercises that you would never have dreamed of trying before. Try some of the sexual stimulation. Try thinking your sexuality through. It's all in private—nobody else has to know.

Except that they *will* know—when you find the man you want, and the sexual relationship that's always been yours for the taking, and the happiness that has always been your reward.

Remember that in sex, as well as anything else, you have to make your own luck, and this is how you can make yours.

TWO

Quiz: How Does Your Sex Life Shape Up?

This quiz will tell you just what's missing in your sex life—and what certainly *isn't*! It's been compiled from a questionnaire in which I asked 250 single women all across the United States what they wanted most out of sex, what they weren't getting, and what they *were* getting but didn't want.

Although it's been designed mainly for single women, married women or women who are living with a long-term lover will find it equally profitable. Sometimes it's more of a problem having a man who doesn't satisfy you than having no man at all.

1. I have sexual intercourse as often as I wish......
.... YES/NO
2. Mostly, my sex life is physically satisfying.........
.... YES/NO
3. Mostly, my sex life is emotionally satisfying......
.... YES/NO
4. I fantasize about a more exciting sex life ....
.... YES/NO
5. I have never met a man who knows how to satisfy me in bed .... YES/NO
6. My experience of sex has been generally good..
.... YES/NO

7. I don't think I know enough about sex and sexual technique.................................... YES/NO
8. I haven't had an orgasm for over a month........ .... YES/NO
9. I haven't had an orgasm for over six months .... YES/NO
10. I haven't dated a man who attracts me for over a month.................................... YES/NO
11. I haven't dated a man who attracts me for over six months .... YES/NO
12. I think I know how to please men in bed......... .... YES/NO
13. I would consider doing new things in bed to please a man .... YES/NO
14. I like the idea of oral sex..................... YES/NO
15. I always carry condoms with me.......... YES/NO
16. I would be too shy to tell a man what really turns me on.. YES/NO
17. I think it is wrong to dress sexily to attract men .... YES/NO
18. I would never allow a man to inspect me sexually .... YES/NO
19. I enjoy masturbation .... YES/NO
20. Masturbation is an admission of sexual failure .... YES/NO
21. I think I would enjoy a vibrator........... YES/NO
22. I would never consider sex on a first date......... .... YES/NO
23. I enjoy kissing .... YES/NO
24. I enjoy men fondling my breasts.......... YES/NO
25. I would do a striptease for a man I liked.......... .... YES/NO
26. I think that it is wrong for women to change their personality for the sake of attracting or keeping a man.. YES/NO
27. I think everything except straight sexual intercourse is perverted .... YES/NO

28. I would never swallow a man's semen .... YES/NO
29. I would be embarrassed to inspect myself sexually .... YES/NO
30. I am not sure how to handle a man's penis properly .... YES/NO
31. I would never have sex without being in love ... . YES/NO
32. I would consider dressing up in sexy underwear to arouse a man .... YES/NO
33. I am not a particularly sexually attractive person .... YES/NO
34. I would never consider a one-night stand .... YES/NO
35. I don't particularly care what men look like, provided they are wealthy.......................... YES/NO
36. I would consider a sexual partner of a different faith .... YES/NO
37. I have sexual fantasies that are too crude to tell anyone .... YES/NO
38. I would enjoy a man's finger in my anus .... YES/NO
39. I would never make love to more than one man at once .... YES/NO
40. Sexual relationships are for life .... YES/NO
41. I am frightened that I would be unable to satisfy a man in bed...................................... YES/NO
42. I don't like looking at myself naked..... YES/NO
43. I would find it hard to share my bed/bathroom/life with a man...................... YES/NO
44. Sometimes I think I would do anything, just to feel a man's penis inside me................ YES/NO
45. I think about sex a lot (more than three or four times a day)... YES/NO
46. I find it difficult to show a man I'm sexually interested in him without feeling whorish......... .... YES/NO

47. I perform acts of self-stimulation which I would never describe to anybody .... YES/NO
48. Men are interested only in having sex with me. .... YES/NO
49. I have an unusually strong sexual appetite .... YES/NO
50. I have been too emotionally damaged to consider new sexual relationships .... YES/NO
51. I think I am responsible for the breakup of all or most of my previous sexual relationships .... YES/NO
52. I like sex that involves a certain degree of pain .... YES/NO
53. I think men use me as a toilet .... YES/NO
54. No man would ever seriously be interested in having a long-term sexual relationship with me .... YES/NO
55. I don't think that there is any hope of my having a happy sex life .... YES/NO
56. I would never consider advertising for a partner in a magazine .... YES/NO
57. I expect a man to take control in a sexual relationship .... YES/NO
58. I wouldn't like any man to know how lonely I feel .... YES/NO
59. I think all pornography is disgusting ... YES/NO
60. I prefer lovemaking in the dark .... YES/NO
61. If I knew more about sex I would be a better lover .... YES/NO
62. I am not interested in learning how to please a man sexually .... YES/NO
63. I think I need to know more about pleasing men sexually .... YES/NO

Scoring will take you just a few moments. If you answered "Yes" to the following questions, score 1 *red* point: 1, 2, 3, 6, 12, 13, 14, 15, 19, 21, 23, 24, 25,

26, 32, 36, 37, 38, 45, 47, 49. If you answered "Yes" to all of them, you would have scored 21 *red* points.

If you answered "Yes" to the following questions, score 1 *yellow* point: 4, 8, 10, 16, 20, 22, 28, 30, 31, 33, 34, 39, 40, 41, 44, 46, 51, 58, 60, 61, 63. If you answered "Yes" to all of them, you would have scored 21 *yellow* points.

If you answered "Yes" to the following questions, score 1 *blue* point: 5, 7, 9, 11, 17, 18, 27, 29, 35, 42, 43, 48, 50, 52, 53, 54, 55, 56, 57, 59, 62. If you answered "Yes" to all of them, you would have scored 21 *blue* points.

So what does this quiz tell you about the current status of your sex life? Although it is by no means a fully comprehensive questionnaire, it can give you a very clear profile of how you feel about sex and men and about the prospect of looking for a partner.

If you scored more than 15 red points, then you're something of a red-hot lover. You're interested in sex, you're not afraid to look for sexual satisfaction, and you're prepared to enter into a sexual relationship with enthusiasm and commitment. You accept the desirability of discussing sex and learning about erotic techniques in order to improve your lovemaking.

Most importantly, you consider yourself an equal partner in your sexual relationships with men—a partner with her own needs and desires—but with her own responsibilities in the achievement of successful and fulfilling sex.

If you scored fewer than 15 red points, then you're still a very erotic and adventurous person, but you do tend to think twice before abandoning your inhibitions and letting yourself go. You're passionate, giving, and interested in fulfilling yourself emotionally and physically, but there are definite limits to your sexual liberality. In other words, when you're in bed with a man, you always keep one metaphorical foot on the floor.

If you scored more yellow points than red points, then you are showing yourself that you have strong needs and strong desires, but that you are quite shy in potentially sexual situations and that your sexual confidence doesn't match your sexual appetite. In fact, you are embarrassed about admitting openly that you do have such a thing as a sexual appetite. You have a very strong need to be loved, but you are cautious about committing yourself physically, and you are concerned that you might jeopardize your intimate relationships with men because you don't know enough about sex or sexual techniques.

If you have more than 15 yellow points, it is clear that your sexual inhibitions are causing real difficulties in your emotional life. With the help of this book, and with the help of your friends, you should try to pinpoint all of those aspects of sex that make you feel anxious or embarrassed. You will be amazed how easy it is to overcome most sexual problems once you have actually faced up to them.

Try to analyze *why* you feel inhibited about sex. You don't need to go to an expensive psychoanalyst to recall those critical moments in your life when your opinions about sex were first formed, and you don't need months of therapy in order to deal with them. I have been talking to men and women about sex and sexual problems for 25 years, and I have very rarely come across a sexual difficulty that a couple or an individual doesn't have the strength and the character to sort out by themselves.

In fact, without realizing it you have started to sort out your sexual inhibitions already, simply by truthfully saying that you have scored so many yellow points. They say that a problem shared is a problem halved; but you can equally say that a problem confronted is a problem that's well on the way to not being a problem any longer.

What if you've scored more blue points than yellow points? In that case, your sexual inhibitions are compounded by your unwillingness to let go of them. Your perception of men is suspicious and occasionally hostile—either because of the way you were introduced to sex or because of a negative sexual experience with a man. This negative sexual experience might range from something as inconsequential as the man's inability to sustain a full erection when he made love to you or your inability to reach an orgasm, to sexual bullying, humiliation, or rape.

In the preparation of this book, I talked to a single woman of 23 whose first lover had insisted on sex whenever and wherever he felt like it, and who had beaten her if she showed any signs of resistance. She had never known any other kind of sexual relationship, and she had quickly grown to assume that this raping and beating was normal. When she discovered that other women's lovers didn't hit them and humiliate them every day, she was astonished. "It was like waking up after a nightmare."

If you have scored more than 15 blue points, then you ought to be asking yourself *why* you feel so defensive about sex. Your answer might be very uncomplicated, such as, "I just don't like sex very much." Don't leave it at that, though. Ask yourself what it is that you don't like. Is it the fact that you've never enjoyed it in the past? Is it the lack of control? Are you embarrassed about showing your naked body?

Everybody varies in their attitudes toward sex and sexual pleasure. Some women adore pornography while others find it totally repulsive. Some women enjoy sex every single day, others are content with two or three times a month. There is no such thing as "normal" sexual behavior.

What there is, however, is personal satisfaction. And if you've finished up with a high score of blue points, then the chances are that you are not being sexually fulfilled. I'm not saying that you're unfulfilled in comparison with other women. You're unfulfilled in comparison with your own needs and your own sexual potential.

Fortunately, the strongest sexual inhibitions are often the easiest to identify and to cure. During the course of preparing this book, I was in fairly constant contact with Eve, a 33-year-old beautician from Philadelphia who had been virtually celibate for over six years after the breakup of her marriage.

Eve filled out a very much longer questionnaire than the one printed above, and her sexual inhibitions were quite alarming.

It turned out that she had been *very* passionate and *very* interested in sex when she was younger. Her first lover had been a man seven years her senior who had introduced her (gently, she said) to all kinds of sexual variations—oral sex, mutual masturbation, anal sex, outdoor sex, a little bit of mild bondage, wet sex.

Unfortunately her husband had been brought up in a household where sex was never mentioned, and when it came to sex, he was very repressed. He found Eve's bedtime demands to be more than he could deal with and retaliated by calling her a slut and a whore.

"The worst moment came after Gary had been out playing golf one afternoon. He came back and took a shower and I committed the sin of sins—I took off my clothes and joined him in the shower stall. He was angry at first, but then I washed his back for him and soaped his chest and he seemed to enjoy it. I thought I was actually making some headway, if you know what I mean. We were kissing and caressing, and his cock was real hard, and I was getting really turned on. I began to feel *happy* about our sexual relationship for the first time since we'd been together.

"I guided his hand down between my legs, so that

he could feel me. He seemed to like that, too. He slipped his finger up inside my cunt, and everything was going fantastically. But then I made the mistake of doing something that had always driven Rickie (my first boyfriend) really crazy with desire. I pissed over Gary's hand, and kissed him as I pissed. It ran down our legs, all hot and warm, and I thought: This is going to turn him on like you wouldn't believe.

"But he went ape. He screamed at me, 'What are you doing, that's disgusting! That's totally disgusting!' He took the nailbrush and he started to scrub at his hand as if I'd given him some kind of terrible disease. He made me feel filthy and awful and cheap. He demoralized me completely.

"After that, we didn't make love for about a month. Gary even told me that he'd talked to a psychiatrist about me, because he thought I had some kind of infantile fixation with urine. How could I explain that I pissed in his hand because pissing is sexy—at least between two people who really love each other?

"Eventually—and this was the worst thing—I actually began to believe that what I had done was disgusting. Gary convinced me that I was depraved and dirty, that I was some kind of whore. In fact, he made me feel worse than a whore. We stopped making love altogether, and I think that Gary preferred it that way.

"It wasn't until I filled out your questionnaire that I began to say to myself—hold on here, is this *really* the way I feel about sex? And it wasn't. It was the way that *Gary* felt about sex. He had completely subjugated me. Maybe he was jealous about my previous life and wanted me to feel guilty about it. Maybe he just couldn't come to terms with his sexuality, period. But *he* was the one who needed the therapy, not me. I *liked* sex, until I met him. I was happy the way I was.

"It was like coming out of amnesia. Once I remembered that I used to be happy, Gary's influence over me was completely broken. With one bound, I was free!

"I think my experience is very, very common. I think far too many women allow themselves to be influenced by men because they're afraid of being alone, afraid of having to take care of themselves.

"And the trouble is, there's a whole lot of men out there who don't know dick about sex, if you'll pardon my language. They're repressive, they're aggressive, and too many women are having to spend their whole lives saying yes, nossir, three-bags-full sir, accepting crude and ignorant and clumsy sex, when there is real *passion* to be had, real excitement. My advice to all women is to go piss in their man's hand tonight . . . and if that doesn't turn them on, then pack your bags and leave."

I wouldn't actually recommend that you follow Eve's advice to the letter. There are far less provocative ways of sorting out a sexual relationship that's gone off the rails. But, on the whole, she has some sensible words to say, and I know from experience that there are countless thousands of women who never get to experience the full pleasure of sex because their partners are inexperienced, inhibited, or just plain ignorant.

To be ignorant about sex is not a crime. Sex is a complex subject, both psychologically and physiologically (mind and body), and we are discovering new things about sex every day. But what *is* unforgiveable is to have a closed mind about sex, to say, *I don't like this and I never will, I'm not trying this and I never will.* A man who refuses to educate himself sexually is guilty of a serious offense—the offense of depriving himself and his partner of pleasure and fulfilment and happiness.

Similarly, a woman who allows a sexually ignorant man to dominate her life is guilty of shortchanging herself both physically and emotionally. If you're sexually alone because you don't have a man, or if you're sexually alone because you *do* have a man and he doesn't know how to please you, then think about this: These years will never come back again, these years when you're bright and brilliant and right in your sexual prime.

See how many points you've scored in this questionnaire and then make up your mind that from now on, your love life is going to be red, sizzling hot—just the way you want it!

THREE

Single But Very, Very Sexy

"My parents just can't understand that I *want* to stay single!"

That was the protest of 27-year-old Karen, a pretty, dark-haired artist from San Francisco. Karen graduated from art college at the age of 23 as a potter, and set up her own successful pottery in Sausalito.

"I like men and I like sex, but I also like space. One day I want to settle down with a man and have children. But I don't want to do it yet—and I don't want to do it until I find the *right* man."

And here's Alma, 38, a handsome natural blonde from St. Louis, currently making her living as an in-store beautician. "I was married, I was divorced. Now I'm single again. I'd love to have a man around the house. I'd love to have a man in my bed every night. But not at any price. I'm not going through that again—once in a lifetime is quite enough!"

Today, there are millions of women leading the single life (a) because they haven't found a man they want to marry; or (b) because they don't want to get married until they've fulfilled their career ambitions; or (c) because they're divorced or separated and haven't yet found a new partner.

Let's not beat around the bush—for these women, finding regular and fulfilling sex is a serious problem. Perhaps it wasn't quite as difficult before AIDS became such a menace. There was always the option of the singles bar pickup, or the casual acquaintance met at a party. But these days, the threat of HIV infection is such that a woman can't even trust a man she has known for years and years.

Single women find themselves the victims not only of social attitudes that *still* favor couples, but of a worldwide epidemic that makes casual sex the next most dangerous pastime after Russian roulette.

Their need for loving company, and sometimes their desperation, can be seen in magazines and newspapers all over the nation. And these are all genuine personals, taken from quality mass-market publications.

- "Pretty, petite, sensual 28-year-old with great legs, SWF, educated professional, true romantic, adventurous and playful. I enjoy dancing, travel, theater, fine dining, picnics, biking, hugs, etc. I believe variety is the spice of life. You should be a handsome successful gentleman who is appreciative, has a great sense of humor and enjoys sports. Preferably between 5'9" and 6'1", nonsmoker. Letter, phone, photo."
- "Very attractive, energetic, engaging, slender, blonde SWF MD, 36, multifaceted background blending Northeastern sophistication, Southern charm and Midwestern values. Enjoys cosmopolitan and country travel, MFA, tennis, dancing and culinary pleasures. Seeking accomplished, well-educated, cultured, kind, clean-cut gentleman who is active and reflective; for committed relationship, valuing affection, humor, communication and friendship."
- "Sensual Mediterranean beauty—with brains— seeks 35ish handsome blue-eyed artsy educated gentleman. A genuine and genuinely good human being with lots o' lasting Leo love, laughter and good food to share. Into gardening, libraries and

fast cars. Looking forward to great conversation, romantic evenings, and a willingness to laugh at life's funny moments. Unretouched photos, please."

- "Lovely and lonely, this pretty, slim, expressive woman, '40s, seeks sensuous, adventurous, unpretentious, permanent partner."

In the course of researching this book, I contacted 50 women, all across the country, who had placed personal advertisements in the hope of finding a man.

Their needs and responses were remarkably similar. They were looking more than anything else for companionship—and everything that companionship implies. That is, security, friendship, affection, decisiveness—a man who could give their life some social stability.

Whatever the achievements of the feminist movement—and there have been many—the fact remains that it is still very difficult for a woman to lead a successful and fulfilling social life on her own. The way in which our social occasions are structured makes it essential for a woman to have an escort or a partner or a lover or a husband. Eating *à deux* in a fashionable restaurant is romantic for a couple; for a single man it's awkward (paperback book propped up on the cruet); for a single woman it's almost intolerable.

Personally, I believe that single women ought to be able to socialize comfortably wherever and whenever they wish. But the reality, regrettably, is very different. All of the single women to whom I spoke while I was preparing this book—and I mean *all*—100 percent— said that at one time or another, they had been approached by a man and asked for sex outright, as if they were a prostitute.

And almost all of them reported that they had encountered extremely hostile responses from married women whenever they attended a social occasion on their own.

Let's take a look, first of all, at those women who say that they have never found the right partner. Sometimes it's clear that they really haven't.

Jane, a 25-year-old insurance broker from Seattle, said, "I had a three-year affair with my high school sweetheart, Carl. Everybody thought that we were going to get married and live happily ever after, but not long after we were engaged my sister and her husband asked me if I wanted to take a three-week vacation in Europe with her. I said sure, I jumped at the chance, and Carl didn't mind. But that three-week vacation opened my eyes. I saw Paris, I saw London, I saw Vienna. I met all kinds of different men. Some of them were romantic, some of them were rude. In Paris, a man called Jean-Claude asked me to dinner. He was doing some legal work for my brother-in-law, something to do with international trade. Afterwards, he took me back to his apartment and made love to me. It was just like a movie.

"There was classical music playing, and the sound of someone arguing in French on the other side of the apartment building. Jean-Claude wasn't handsome but you couldn't say he was ugly, either. He was kind of *battered*, you know, as if he had really lived life. And he had this long hair, streaked with gray, and this bent nose, and eyes that could look right down inside your soul, and inspect your panties from the inside. He was the total opposite of Carl.

"Carl was tall and tanned and completely perfect. Kind of like Superman, if you know what I mean! He believed in truth, justice, and the American way. Whereas Jean-Claude was dissolute and rude and evasive and *so-o-o* romantic. I didn't believe a word he said but he said I was like a mermaid that he had found washed up on the banks of the Seine. He gave me

Chateau Talbot to drink, which is a rich red wine that made my head spin. I remember the name because I kept the label. He said that mermaids have oysters instead of genitals; but if a man can pry them open, he will always be rewarded by the moistest, most succulent feast imaginable.

"I think I was pretty drunk. I *know* I was pretty drunk. I lay back on this couch and Jean-Claude knelt beside me and kissed me—my face, my hair, my neck. He was in full evening dress—wing-collar, black tie, tuxedo, everything. He said he hated the word 'tuxedo,' it was so American-vulgar. In France, they called a tuxedo 'le smoking'. Doesn't that make your head spin? 'Le smoking', I love it. I was certainly smoking that evening.

"He lifted my evening dress over my thighs. He didn't touch my breasts. I was wearing pantyhose and I never wear panties with pantyhose. He said, 'I can see your oyster in its net. It is glistening with passion.' What he meant was that my pussy was wet. He made me totally delirious.

"He dragged down my pantyhose with his teeth. Can you imagine that! With his teeth! I dug my hands into his hair. He smelled of lavender and cigars. Such an old-fashioned smell, I can smell it now. He tugged at my pubic hair with his teeth, and then he ran the tip of his tongue all the way down my pussy, from the top to the bottom, and poked the tip of his tongue into my asshole. I mean, nobody had ever done that to me before. Nothing like that. Carl wouldn't have dreamed of going down on me—jocks didn't go down on girls. But here was this handsome, battered-looking guy in full evening dress, prodding his tongue up my bare asshole.

"I felt like the world was caving in. He licked around and around my asshole, sometimes dipping the tip of his tongue right into it. It felt wet and shivery and so weird. Then he started licking my pussy. His tongue slid down one lip and slid up the other. He touched my clitoris, but only lightly. Then he was running his tongue back down again, until he found my peehole, and he started licking that, too. His tongue went right inside my pussy, and he *sucked* me, he *drank* me, like he really wanted me, he couldn't get enough of me. I thought: This man doesn't just want to fuck me, he doesn't just want to make me feel better. I turn him on. He wants to eat me.

"He flicked my clitoris with his tongue, very very lightly, very fast, so that it began to feel as if it was ten times its normal size, all swelled up and tingly. Then he ran his tongue down my pussy again, exploring every single crevice, as if he wanted to know me totally, licking and sucking all the time. Then he went back to my clitoris, and I had another surge, and another incredible feeling, like I was Mount Saint Helen's or something, about to erupt.

"He licked me and licked me, and I didn't realize that I was about to come until a few seconds before it happened. I had this tense feeling in my back—almost a pain. My pelvis was rigid. I opened my legs wider and wider, and caught hold of Jean-Claude's hair, and forced his face deeper and deeper into my pussy. He licked quicker and quicker. His tongue tip was really dancing. I was so wet that I had soaked the brocade on the sofa. He slid one finger into my pussy, and slowly swirled it around, a kind of a slow, spiral movement, and that was something I'd never felt before. Then he slid another finger into my asshole, and began to tug that, too.

"I had experienced orgasms before, but I had never experienced an orgasm like this. I simply wasn't in control. I don't know whether I shouted out loud or not. But I felt like worlds had collided. This wasn't the earth moving, this was the universe faltering, the whole damned universe. My hips wouldn't stop bouncing up and down for about five minutes.

"Do you know what I did in return? I opened the fly of his evening pants and took out his cock. It was very big and dark, and the head was almost purple, like a plum. I sucked it hard, and took it halfway down my throat. I felt like I wanted to swallow it, to choke on it. I sucked it and I rubbed it, and then he suddenly said something French—maybe '*mon Dieu*,' something like that—and my whole mouth filled up with his sperm.

"I'd never taken a man's sperm in my mouth before. Carl hadn't really been into oral sex, remember. But I was determined to relish it. I opened my mouth wide so that sperm ran down my chin, and then I licked my lips and swallowed, and sucked his cock until there was nothing left.

"That experience changed my life. I saw Jean-Claude only once after that, in a café on the Champs Elysees. He was in a hurry, very distracted. I looked at his face and thought, my God, that man has licked my vagina. That man's tongue tip (from which he's just picking a shred of tobacco) has probed up my asshole, the most private part of my body. Yet now he's sitting here, and he's anxious to leave, he wants to leave me?

"But then I understood why. He was a single man, he was frightened of love. He was *capable* of love, for sure—he was *capable* of loyalty. But he wanted to be free. Today *my* pussy; tomorrow somebody else's. I understood why he needed his freedom and why it was frightening, too. What happens when you grow old and unattractive? What happens when the girls look at you and laugh?

"I also understood something else. I understood that I was making a serious mistake in thinking that I *had* to marry Carl—that it was carved in Roman lettering in tablets of stone. I didn't love him. I hadn't been loyal to him. He was nothing more than the easiest option. If we got married, everybody at home would say 'Isn't it wonderful?' But we'd be sitting in front of a divorce lawyer before we knew it. I had a man friend who wore his best pants to court, to attend his divorce hearing, and while he was listening to his wife's lawyer he found rice in his cuffs. The last time he'd worn those pants was on their wedding day. I didn't want anything like that to happen to me.

"I'm still single, but I've dated six or seven men, and I was tempted to settle down with one of them. Tempted—but that was just about as far as it went. I don't think women should be afraid of being choosy. People who are choosy usually have good, long-lasting relationships. I think there's something else, too, which is far more important than being choosy, and that's to have the same goals, the same vision in life; or as near as, damn it.

"And one thing more: flexibility, and the ability to compromise, and sometimes to say you're sorry when you're not really sorry, just for the sake of the ongoing relationship.

"I haven't found a man with whom I'm prepared to compromise; not just yet. Nor a man to whom I can say I'm sorry when I'm not sorry. Remember he has to do the same to me. But I've found two or three men who are caring and sexy and kind, and I've had some very good times, and I've had some very good cocks in my mouth—which is something that never would have happened if I'd married Carl.

"Sometimes I feel lonely. Sometimes I feel scared. Oh, God—supposing I never meet anybody, ever! But most of the time I feel whole, and content. Reasonably whole, and reasonably content. Wouldn't it be *good* though, to wake up one morning and find that Jean-Claude was in bed with me, tonguing my pussy?"

What interested me about Jane was that she was

able to come out with such sound opinions on sex and sexual relationships, even though she was unable to find a man with whom she wanted to start up a long-term affair. It helps a great deal when a couple have "the same goals, the same vision in life." You'd be startled how many relationships I come across in which the man and the woman have almost diametrically opposing ideas about why they're together and what they're trying to achieve.

I talked to a 38-year-old golf pro in Napa, California, who believed that "flexibility is another enormous plus. I believe in standing firm on major ethical principles, but there are times when a little give-and-take can make the difference between a kiss and a hug and a serious row. Saying sorry now and again never hurt anybody, even if you're sorry only because you had an argument, and not because you're prepared to admit that you're wrong."

Jane is typical of a great many young single women who (because of their early sexual maturity and because of their attractiveness) form steady relationships with boys at high-school age. Particularly when they're living in small, relatively stable communities, such as agricultural towns in the Midwest, or ethnically concentrated suburbs of major cities, they find after a very short while that they've been imprisoned by the expectations of their friends and their parents, and that escaping from this high-school "engagement" is very, very difficult indeed. You know the kind of situation I'm talking about: "Oh . . . but we always expected you to marry the Greenbaum boy . . ."

Most men and women, however, make much better marriage partners when they've had a few years of sexual and emotional experience. It may be highly controversial to suggest it—and, of course, there will always be notable exceptions to the rule—but in my opinion nobody should even think about marriage until they're 27 or over.

If people were to wait just two or three years more before they considered marriage, there would be fewer mistakes, fewer divorces, fewer single-parent families. There would also be fewer lonesome people trying to find a partner in a society that offers very little sympathy to those who have failed to find a soulmate, or to those who have loved and lost.

While I was preparing this book, I talked to scores of men and women who had advertised in magazines and newspapers for partners, and I cannot remember a single one of them who was anything but warm, pleasant, caring, and attractive. They didn't all look like models, and some of them could have thought more carefully about the way they dressed and the way they presented themselves. But, on the whole, there was nothing to distinguish them from the most successful of lovers that I have ever come across.

No—I tell a lie. There was one quality that tended to be lacking in single or separated people. Our old friend, sexual self-confidence.

Any woman who hasn't yet been able to find herself a lover is bound to question her sexual attractiveness and her ability to arouse men. The same goes for any woman who has been divorced, or who has suffered the breakup of a long-term sexual relationship. No matter how much you tell yourself that *he* had no taste, that *he* was in the wrong . . . even if you hate his guts and you never want even to *think* about him ever again . . . the fact remains that you will always have doubts about yourself. You will always ask yourself, *Was it me?* And the longer you remain unattached, the more your sexual self-confidence will be eroded.

In just a minute, you'll see that no woman needs to suffer from a lack of sexual self-confidence (a) because there is no case, *ever*, where a lack of sexual self-confidence is justified; and (b) because a lack of sexual self-confidence is so easy to overcome.

But the fact is that many single women *do* feel unsure of their sexuality, and this unsureness very often adds to their difficulties in forming intimate relationships.

To be brutally frank, a lack of sexual self-confidence can actually turn men off. It manifests itself in all kinds of different ways, but the effect is almost always the same. It drives away the very person you're more interested in trying to attract. You want them (oh, how much you want them!) but somehow you always manage to say or do the wrong thing and put them off.

Now, why do you *do* this? Are you a masochist, or what? Do you really want to stay lonesome and unloved for the rest of your life, or do you want an exciting, erotic, and highly satisfying relationship, whether it leads to marriage or not?

You don't have to tick either answer. I know which one you want. Because that's what almost every woman wants.

Here's Emma, 34, a library supervisor from Houston, Texas: "I was divorced when I was 30. My first husband was what you might call my high-school sweetheart. His name was Gene and he was very tall and handsome and he was a brilliant football player. If you'll excuse me sounding vain, I was one of the most glamorous girls in school—the blue-eyed blonde with the well-filled sweater. We kind of made a natural pair. Everybody assumed that we would get married and that's what we did.

"It never occurred to anybody—not even to us—that Gene and I didn't have anything remotely in common. We got along fine at school, because it was all football and listening to music and cruising and hanging out, but once we were married it didn't take me longer than three weeks to realize how dumb we'd been. Or *I'd* been, anyway. Gene seemed to like it. He had some-body to wash and cook for him, somebody to have sex with, whenever he wanted it. But we hardly ever spoke. Now that we didn't go to classes together, now that we didn't meet our friends during recess, we had nothing to say to each other.

"I've always been interested in modern American writing, like Richard Brautigan and Ellen Gilchrist and people like that. I tried to get Gene to read some of their stories but all it did was make him angry. He accused me of trying to make him look stupid. I didn't think he was stupid. I *never* thought he was stupid. But he wasn't interested in anything else but football and cars.

"What really broke up our marriage, though, was our sex life. The sad part about it was, Gene was so physi-cally attractive. He had a fantastic physique—broad shoulders, muscly chest, narrow hips, and one of those tight, hard rounded bottoms that most women could absolutely die for. He had a huge cock, too, even when it was soft. His jeans used to bulge out so much that one of my friends asked me if he padded his shorts with handkerchiefs.

"But he treated sex like a workout. He would climb on top of me, open my legs, force his cock into me, ready or not, and then proceed to do eighty push-ups until he ejaculated. Then he immediately climbed out of bed, took a shower, and spent the rest of the evening reading *Football Forecast* or *Muscular Development*.

"I'm not saying that Gene didn't ever arouse me when he made love to me, but I always ended up feel-ing frustrated and disappointed, because he simply had no idea that I was supposed to be satisfied, too . . . not just in bed, but every which way.

"I tried real hard to encourage him to make our sex life more varied. One early morning, after he'd come back from jogging, I took off my nightshirt and got into the shower with him. He argued at first, and said he needed to take his shower alone, it was part of his routine. But I kissed him and caressed him. Then I knelt down and started kissing his cock. He got a huge hard-on. I sucked him and licked him and gave his balls a real tongue-bath. I started to rub him with my hand, too.

"He was getting real turned on. He leaned back against the side of the shower stall, and his thighs were all tensed up, and his cock was standing out like a tree trunk. It was the first time that I'd really felt that I was in charge of our lovemaking, that *I* was making it happen, rather than him. I knelt up, and took his cock into my mouth as deep as I could, and gave him long, slow sucks, and rolled my tongue all around him. His cock was huge, and I could feel the slippery juice coming out of him. He was so tense I thought his muscles were going to crack. But then he suddenly seized hold of my hair, and gripped it tight, and rammed his cock even harder into my mouth, in and out, in and out, and I realized that he was using my mouth just as another hot, wet hole to masturbate in. He didn't care if I wanted to do it this way. He didn't care if I was enjoying it. All he wanted to do was to get his rocks off, which he did. I tilted my head back so that his cock slipped out of my mouth, but at the same time he climaxed, and he shot sperm all over my face.

"He was still gripping my hair with his left hand, but he took hold of his cock in his right hand, and slowly used it to massage his sperm all over my face, all around my mouth, all over my cheeks, all over my forehead.

"The way he did it was really macho and careless, but it still could have turned me on if he had done it as foreplay. I mean, I don't mind a man pretending to be rough now and again. It's exciting, so long as he follows it up with with lovemaking, or some way of giving me satisfaction. He could have taken me out of the shower and given me oral sex. He could have masturbated me with his fingers. *Anything,* so long as I got some satisfaction out of our lovemaking, too.

"But all he said was, 'That was great,' and stepped out of the shower, and toweled himself dry, and started to dress.

"I came out of that shower all wet, and aroused, and with my face plastered in sperm. I said, 'Let's go to bed.' But Gene said, 'No way, I have to meet my insurance broker at eleven. Anyway, what do you want to go to bed for? That was great, in the shower. Really great!' And he walked out, and left me.

"Can you imagine how that made me feel? 'That was great, in the shower. Really great!' Maybe for him, but not for me. For the first time since I was about 15 years old, I masturbated. I went naked into the breakfast room and I took out this enormous green candle from the drawer where we keep all the paper napkins. I lay on the couch, and I fantasized that I was being seduced by a handsome alien from another planet, like Gene only green, with a massive green cock. I guess it sounds ridiculous, but I wanted to feel that I was being seduced by somebody who was interested in me, somebody who was curious about me, somebody who wanted to find out what excited me.

"I slowly rubbed my clitoris with my fingers, around and around. I was quite juicy already, from making love with Gene. Then I stretched open my legs very, very wide and pushed this enormous green candle into my vagina, as far as it would go, and a little further. When I looked down, all I could see was my hairy vaginal lips stretched wide open, and about an inch of this emerald green candle sticking out of me.

"I fucked myself. I did it slowly and luxuriously, and enjoyed every moment of it. I knew that I was only making love to an imaginary alien, but I didn't care.

At least I was being touched and fucked and somebody cared what I felt like, even if it was only me.

"Gene never realized that a woman has to have her clitoris stimulated before she can reach an orgasm. I tried to tell him once, tried to show him how to do it, but he pulled his hand away and got all irritable and upset.

"At least, when I was masturbating, I knew exactly how I liked to have my clitoris rubbed and tugged. I had the first orgasm then that I'd experienced in years . . . and it hit me so hard that I was breathless. I lay on my side on that couch for almost five minutes, with that candle right up inside me, shaking and gasping and trembling.

"I suppose I knew then in my heart of hearts that our marriage was over, although I didn't want it to be. I know that Gene and I were completely mismatched, but I was still fond of him, and I was still proud when we walked into a party together and all the women went goggle-eyed. All the same, I used to think to myself: If only you knew how unexciting this man is when it comes to bedtime!

"I did everything I could think of to make him more adventurous in bed, to make him understand that *I* had needs, too. I dressed up in sexy underwear, with a G-string and garter belt and black fishnet stockings, but all he said was, 'Where are you going? A costume party?' I opened the door for him naked when he came back from work, and all he said was, 'Get dressed, for God's sake, you'll catch your death.' No matter what I did or what I suggested, he always ended up angry. He didn't understand that I wasn't criticizing the lovemaking that he *was* giving me, I just wanted more of it. I just wanted him to realize that he aroused me, but he had to fulfill me, too."

Although Emma now sounds reasonably confident when she talks about the failure of her sexual relationship with Gene, she went through a lengthy period of increasing despair and depression, and—wrongly but quite understandably—she began to blame herself for his lack of interest in her.

"I began to think that it must be my fault, that I wasn't attractive enough, that I wasn't sexy enough, that I wasn't any good in bed."

It took Emma a long time—nearly two years—fully to recover her sexual self-esteem. The problem of sexual self-doubt almost always starts a vicious downward spiral, and it takes a considerable amount of strength and courage to overcome it.

Because she had such a low opinion of her attractiveness and her sexuality, Emma actively avoided getting involved in new relationships with men. She began to feel lonely and emotionally isolated, and even when she *did* meet a man she liked, she almost always kept him at arm's length with a combination of defensiveness, cynicism, and self-criticism. It was what I call the "Why-would-you-want-to-date-anyone-like-me?" syndrome.

You know how the conversation goes:

> "Why would you want to date anyone like me?"
> "Because you're pretty."
> "No, I'm not. I'm totally ordinary."
> "You're not ordinary. You're terrific looking."
> "You're just saying that."

And so on and so on, until the man gets tired of arguing.

The single most important skill that a single woman can ever develop in starting a new relationship with a man is to learn to accept his compliments with obvious pleasure and good grace. If you persist in denying that you're attractive, you're as good as saying that he has no taste, and that he's an idiot for liking you. Either that, or you'll give him the impression that you enjoy flattery so much that you want to hear very much more before you'll be satisfied.

I know that it's very easy to slip into the habit of picking holes in yourself, especially when you're shy or embarrassed or you've lost your confidence in your own sexual attractiveness. Emma said, "Every time a man said, 'I love your hair,' I always used to say, 'I hate it. The stylist made a complete mess of it.' Every time a man said, 'You have a fabulous figure,' I always used to say 'I'm top heavy. I'm thinking of having a reduction.' They couldn't say one nice word to me without my snapping back. It was only because I was embarrassed about being complimented, and I was frightened of getting myself involved with somebody new."

Although the reality was that her marriage had broken up because of Gene's failure to satisfy her, Emma was sure that she was no good at all at attracting and pleasing a man in bed. Her divorce had been emotionally painful and socially humiliating ("How could you possibly let a hunk like *that* get away!) and she wasn't at all anxious to repeat the experience.

Emma's first step on the road to recovery was to learn to perceive herself as a whole and independent person and not (as she had been ever since her high school days) a decorative appendage to Gene, or indeed to any other man.

"I felt confused and aggrieved and lonely, and there were plenty of times when I wished that Gene and I hadn't divorced. I kept thinking to myself: If only I'd been more a woman, if only I'd been more sexually expert, I could have shown him how to please me. I accepted all of the blame, all of the guilt. Apart from that, I felt as though I was only one-half of something that was broken, like a single book-end or a left-hand stereo speaker or a lost glove."

Our society is still largely a society of couples, even if

those couples are much-divorced and much-remarried. That's why so many single or divorced or separated women mistakenly perceive themselves, in Emma's words, as "a left-hand stereo speaker," useless without a right-hand complement.

But Emma was lucky in finding not a man but a single woman who gave her a new view on her sexuality. At an art gallery opening in Houston, she met Bea, 28, a striking and successful painter. They got talking and a friendship developed, during the course of which Bea helped to restore almost all of Emma's sexual self-assuredness.

"Bea told me that she adored men and she loved sex. At first, she frightened me, because she seemed so sure of herself. She seemed to know exactly what she wanted and to go for it—and that included men! But when we got to talking, I gradually realized that she wasn't really aggressive. She had the same anxieties about the same things as I did. She had the same butterflies in her stomach when she talked to men. But what she didn't have was the fear that I had, that I wouldn't be good enough in bed, that I wasn't sexy, that I wasn't attractive.

"Gradually, I realized what Bea's secret was. It wasn't so much that she was sure of what she wanted, it was the fact that she was sure of *who she was*. She had taken the trouble to get to know herself—her ideas, her ambitions, her social position, her needs, her looks, her sexuality and her body. She had literally sat down and mapped herself out. She knew her abilities and her limitations. She knew what excited her about sex and what turned her off. She knew what her fantasies were and wasn't ashamed of them. She knew what she was looking for when it came to men. But she wasn't hard-and-fast about it. She was always happy to be surprised. Sometimes she surprised herself, by thinking of a sexual fantasy which she had never thought of before, and really turning herself on.

"Once, when she was working on a real big painting, she had the television switched to a baseball game. She's not particularly interested in baseball, but she thought that the excitement of the crowd was so infectious. That night, in bed, she had a fantasy that she was trying to find her seat in a baseball stadium. She was wearing a sweatshirt and a little short pleated skirt, with no panties underneath. She had to push past thirty or forty men, and as she approached, each one of them opened up his fly and took out a huge stiff cock. When she tried to pass by, they pulled her down into their laps, and penetrated her, one after the other, really pulling her down so that their cocks went right up her, and then climaxing, and passing her onto the man sitting in the next seat. By the time she had been pulled down by the tenth man, she had an orgasm, and then it was one orgasm after another, all the way along the line. And all around her the crowd was cheering the game, and there was this immense feeling of excitement, as if the whole crowd knew that she was being fucked, too.

"She reached her seat with thirty men's sperm running down her legs. She said she could feel how hot and aroused she felt! She massaged the sperm all over her thighs and between her legs and everywhere, and took handfuls of it and licked it. She says that in her fantasies sperm tastes like vanilla.

"Then the home team's star hitter came up from the dugout and presented her with his bat. She said he was all dark and sweaty and handsome, and had eyes like John Travolta. I wish I had *her* imagination! She took the bat, and lifted up her skirt, and twisted the bat handle into her vagina, as far as it would go, and worked it up and down, so that he could watch her. Then she took out the bat, and gave it back to him, and licked his sweaty forehead, and told him he was going to win now, for sure, he has going to hit that first ball right out of the park."

Of course, Emma had talked about men with other women, but she had never realized that other women harbored sexual fantasies as graphic and as powerful as any of her own. Neither had she realized that it was not only possible but essential for a single woman to have a sexual identity entirely of her own, quite independent of her sexual identity with a man.

"Bea invited me around one afternoon to her studio, and we got to talking about sex and orgasms and what aroused us most of all. Bea said that hardly any of her lovers had taken the trouble to stimulate her breasts properly. They *liked* her breasts, because she had beautiful big rounded breasts, with really wide nipples; but most of the time her lovers had just fumbled with them a little and then gone hurrying on 'downstairs.' Of course that was pretty much the same experience that I'd had with Gene. He had never taken the trouble to make sure that I was properly aroused. I don't feel the need for an orgasm every single time I make love, and I don't think that many women do. An orgasm isn't the be-all and end-all of lovemaking. But I do feel the need to be wanted, to be loved, to be close, to be highly stimulated. What I used to hate about sex with Gene is that I would be just beginning to get aroused, just beginning to feel that delicious itch, and then it would all be over.

"Bea and I had a couple of glasses of wine that afternoon, and we started to get very affectionate and close. She grasped her breasts through her dress and said, 'I really like them being squeezed like this, strong and slow.' Then she lifted up her dress, and she was naked underneath. She showed me how she liked having her breasts massaged and her nipples twisted and tugged at the same time. She loved that insistent tugging on her nipples.

"She said, 'Here . . . see what it feels like when somebody else does it.' She unbuttoned my blouse, and unfastened my bra, and massaged my breasts in the same way. At first I was shy and cautious about what she was doing, but the sensation was fabulous, and I knew that she wasn't gay. Even if she *had* been, it wouldn't have mattered. She was showing me how to take control of my own responses.

"She took off her dress completely, and then she unbuckled my jeans and undressed me, too. It was strange having another woman take down my panties. I was still feeling shy, but I couldn't help feeling very excited, too, and breathless. Bea led me through to the bedroom, and spread a sheet over the bed. Then she told me to lie back, and she climbed astride me. She opened a bottle of baby oil and poured it onto my breasts. It felt cold at first, and I shivered, but then she started to massage it around and around on my breasts, while she tugged and twisted my nipples around. Nobody had ever lavished that much attention on stimulating my breasts before, not even me, and I was amazed at the fantastically erotic sensation that I began to feel. I suddenly thought to myself: I could have an orgasm just having my breasts massaged like this, without even touching my clitoris.

"Bea smothered baby oil on her own breasts, and then squeezed and pressed and massaged our breasts together. She started to kiss me, little kisses at first, but then deep, deep kisses with her tongue in my mouth.

"I kept wanting her to touch me between my legs, to bring me off, but she went on massaging my breasts and kissing me and running her fingers down my back. I was almost going mad with anticipation by now, I wanted her to touch my clitoris so much. At the same time, I didn't want her to stop caressing my breasts, either. Both of us had stiff nipples, and Bea held her breasts in her hands and rubbed and touched our nipples together.

"I don't know how long this went on, but I was so turned on that I was practically out of my mind. It was then that Bea turned around, and sat on top of me, caressing my thighs and all around my stomach. She parted my thighs, and massaged her breasts in between my legs, her nipples flicking my clitoris. Then she opened up my pussy with her fingers, and licked me.

"Never in the whole of my life had I ever felt anything like that. Bea's tongue tip went everywhere, all wet and warm and wriggly. She licked my anus, around and around. At first I winced because I didn't want her to do it, because I was embarrassed. But she coaxed my anus open with her fingers and poked the tip of her tongue right into it, and the feeling made me shiver all the way down my spine with pleasure.

"Then she slid her tongue into my vagina, and licked all around, this gentle, insistent licking. At last she came to my clitoris, and I could feel her tongue tip literally dancing on it, the feeling was so light.

"She was showing me that I needed gentle, slow foreplay, that I was the kind of woman who took a long time to be stimulated . . . but that when I *was* stimulated I could feel the deepest, most incredible feelings ever. I mean, talk about the earth moving.

"Bea's open vagina was right in front of my face. She didn't do anything to encourage me to stimulate her in return, but I had never seen another woman's sex so close before, and never had the opportunity actually to touch it. I lifted my head and kissed her vaginal lips, a very chaste kiss! Her lips were bright pink and swollen and her vagina was very juicy.

"I kissed her again, and this time I gave her a little lick. I didn't know whether I was going to like the taste. But it was gorgeous, it tasted so sweet. I licked her again, and again, and then she gave a moan and pressed her vagina against my mouth. I took a whole mouthful of her vaginal lips, and wiggled my tongue right up inside her vagina, and it was incredible. I was like exploring my own womanhood, if you can understand what I mean. Until I really looked at it, until I felt it and tasted it, I always thought of a woman's vagina as nothing more than a hole for men to put their cocks in. But in actual fact it's a whole wonderful thing in itself, with just as much shape and identity as a man's penis.

"I licked Bea's clitoris, the same way that she was licking mine. Both of us were panting now, and massaging our bodies and our breasts together. Bea slid two or three fingers into my vagina, to make them slippery, and then slowly inserted one of them into my anus. She kept on lightly licking me, and gently massaging her fingers up inside me, and it was then that I had my orgasm. I couldn't stop it. I didn't even realize that it was coming. I was suddenly lifted up and everything went dark. I didn't realize until Bea told me afterward that I actually screamed as well.

"When it was over, we showered and put on robes and sat on the deck to listen to music and finish the wine. I have to admit that I felt kind of embarrassed about what had happened. But Bea reassured me and put it into context. She said, 'You had to find out what you were really like, sexually. We could have talked about it for hours, but with sex, there's nothing like practical experience.' "

From that day on, Emma began to think of herself with much more sexual self-esteem. "It must have showed, because it wasn't more than a month before I met John at a library wholesaler's cocktail party, and I found that I was able to flirt with him and talk to him with complete confidence. I *knew* what kind of a person I was, sexually. I *knew* that I was capable of giving and receiving great pleasure and excitement.

"John and I dated three or four times. Then he took me back to his house and we cooked a meal together, and drank some champagne, and one thing led to another. John was divorced and he hadn't made love to a woman for over a year, so he started off by being very hurried and anxious.

"But I knew that wasn't the way that either of us was going to get any satisfaction out of making love . . . so I slowed him down and gently encouraged him to make love to me as slowly and as tantalizingly as Bea had. He kissed me, and caressed my breasts, and I showed him how I liked him to stroke my nipples, and gently bite them.

"I spent a lot of time caressing him, too, trying to do for him what he was doing for me. He wanted to put on a condom immediately, but I said no, we're not in a hurry, and I went slithering down between his legs and kissed his cock, and licked it, until it was all slippery with saliva . . . and *then* I rolled a condom on him.

"When he went into me, it was heaven. I didn't have an orgasm that first time we made love, but only because he had a different kind of rhythm than the rhythm I was used to, and he climaxed just a little too soon. I couldn't blame him, he hadn't made love for so long. But he was good, we were both good, and I knew that my lovemaking was going to get better and better from now on."

Emma's lovemaking improved because she had learned so much more about her own sexuality. She had learned that she could be very much better in bed than her marriage to Gene had led her to believe. She was in control of her own sexual responses, in control of her own body, in control of the *pace* of her lovemaking.

The greatest single problem that occurs in modern sexual relationships isn't impotence or frigidity or stress or anything of that kind. The greatest single problem that occurs in modern sexual relationships is exactly the same problem that occurred in our forefathers' sexual relationships—men are much more quickly aroused than women.

I talked to scores of men in the course of preparing this book. With only a very few exceptions, men these days are aware that women need very much more sexual foreplay than they do. They've read their *Forum* magazines and their *Playboy Advisors* and seen so many more sex-instruction books and videos than the men of preceding generations—even the men of the "swinging Sixties" and the "licentious Seventies." They know that their own sexual response can be almost instantaneous, whereas a woman usually needs far more caressing and stimulation before she is anywhere near to reaching a climax.

The trouble is, 83 percent of men agreed with this statement, but only 36 percent of women said that their lovers spent enough time on foreplay. The obvious conclusion has to be that men are aware *in theory* of what their women require. But when it comes to lovemaking in practice, they tend to be impatient and selfish, and not to give woman the foreplay they need.

The sexual selfishness of men is one of several key reasons why so many women shy away from marriage or long-term sexual relationships and prefer to stay single. Lynn, 25, a fashion designer from Seattle, said, "I've been seriously involved with five men since the age of 19, but each time I've ended up feeling dissatisfied. I've said to myself, 'This isn't the man I want to spend the rest of my life with.' Why? Because they're always paying lip service to my satisfaction . . . they're always telling me how much they love me, and how much they want me to be happy, but when it comes down to reality, they just don't do it. They want to fuck me, and that's the beginning and the end of it.

"I know I'm pretty, I know I've got a good figure. But I'm not going to be treated like a sexual Barbie doll for the rest of my life, like I've got nothing in my head except empty plastic. I've made a conscious decision to stay single unless I meet a man who actually treats me like a human being, and so far that hasn't happened."

How did Lynn deal with her day-to-day sexual appetites?

"If you're single, and you live alone, you tend to work very hard and play very hard. I'm usually sitting at my drawing board every night until midnight, working on new accessories or ready-to-wears. On the weekend, I do step aerobics and swim and play squash. I have a good circle of friends; I get invited to parties. Occasionally I meet good-looking men and I have sex.

"But if I feel an immediate urge, then I'm not ashamed to say that I masturbate. It's not the same as making love, by any means. It doesn't have any of the same emotional excitement. It's like sexual cotton candy, all sweetness and fantasy but no substance. I own a vibrator, yes. In fact I own *two* vibrators. But they're not so much penis substitutes as ways of making me feel good. I never think of them as penises, when I put them in. I think of them as inanimate sex-aids, things to give me a good feeling. Let's put it this way: I don't have any illusions about them!

"A woman is a person and every person needs to have control of themselves—their emotions, their sexuality, everything. It's okay to compromise in a sexual relationship—like if one partner prefers a particular position or a particular way of making love—but it's not okay to accept carelessness and second-best. The next man who opens his pants and tries to push his cock into my mouth about five minutes after we've been introduced, that man's going to get some teeth-marks where it really hurts. And the next man who turns over and falls asleep as soon as he's finished making love to me, that man is going to have a glass of ice water poured in his ear."

I talked to dozens of women who feel the same way about being treated by men almost as an unpaid prostitute. Despite the advances that women have made at home, in politics and in the workplace, they are still comparatively unemancipated when it comes to sex. Those women like Lynn who object to being treated in bed like second-class citizens can very often find that they have difficulty in attracting and keeping a sex partner.

As we have seen from Emma's experience, the answer is to acquire sexual self-knowledge and the qualities that come with it—sexual self-esteem and sexual self-control. Once you know all that a modern woman needs to know about sex—how your body responds and what erotic stimulation you need for really exciting and satisfying lovemaking—then you can begin to exert far more influence on the sexual side of your relationships with men.

You'll be surprised at the result. Because more often than not men are equally ignorant about sex and sex technique, even in this so-called enlightened and liberal age. And if you can show them how *you* like to be excited and satisfied, you can improve and intensify *their* experience, too.

Every single woman is single for her own reason. She may want to be free by choice. She may never have met a man whom she feels she wants to marry, or with whom she wants to have a long-term sexual relationship. She may be afraid or unwilling to make the emotional commitment that a long-term sexual relationship demands. She may not want children, whereas she knows that her partner probably will. She may be divorced or separated. She may have suffered an unpleasant first experience with sex and feel wary of repeating it. She may have had a very exciting first experience with sex and feel that it will never be quite so good ever again.

She may actually be married—or already involved in a long-term sexual relationship—but sexually and emotionally *feel* as if she's single. In that case, she may be looking for a radical change in her sex life—a divorce or a separation or a major shakeup of the way in which she and her partner make love.

Whatever *your* reason for being single, you can improve and enjoy your own sexuality very much more. If you want to find a partner, then there are plenty of ways of doing it—ways that are very much safer and more effective than you might think.

First of all, it is essential for you to analyze what it is you really want out of your sex life. Then you will have to decide how you're going to get it. You may find that you have to turn many of your existing fears and prejudices on their heads. For instance, would you advertise for a man in a magazine? Would you go out to dinner with a group of total strangers? Would you travel to a distant city for the sake of starting an intimate relationship?

In order to map out your sexual needs, answer these questions as truthfully and as frankly as you can:

Your Sexual Profile

1. I feel that I have sex (a) not frequently enough; (b) just about frequently enough; (c) too frequently for my liking.
2. I like to have a man around (a) all of the time; (b) some of the time; (c) only now and then.
3. My knowledge of sex is (a) quite extensive; (b) reasonable; (c) not particularly wide.
4. If I felt sexually frustrated, and I had no lover, I would consider masturbating (a) without hesitation; (b) with a certain degree of guilt; (c) never.
5. If I were offered an erotic video I would (a) be eager to see it; (b) be quite curious to see it; (c) refuse it.
6. When it comes to manual stimulation, I could describe (a) exactly how I could be brought to orgasm; (b) vaguely; (c) don't really know.
7. I would consider flirting with a strange man (a) any time; (b) with caution; (c) never.
8. I would dress sexily in order to attract men (a) without hesitation; (b) sometimes; (c) never.
9. When it comes to lovemaking, the man should take complete control (a) never; (b) sometimes; (c) always.
10. I would consider giving a man oral sex (a) at any time; (b) occasionally; (c) never.
11. When a man gives me oral sex I find it (a) very arousing; (b) moderately arousing; (c) unarousing.
12. I would like to try some new sexual positions (a) very much; (b) occasionally; (c) not at all.
13. I would be willing to try the following sexual variations: *Bondage* (a) yes; (b) possibly; (c) never. *Group sex* (a) yes; (b) possibly; (c) never. *Rubberwear* (a) yes; (b) possibly; (c) never. *Out-*

door sex (a) yes; (b) possibly; (c) never. *Wet Sex* (a) yes; (b) possibly; (c) never. *Anal sex* (a) yes; (b) possibly; (c) never.

14. I have sexual fantasies (a) often; (b) from time to time; (c) hardly ever.

15. I find my sexual fantasies (a) very arousing; (b) quite arousing; (c) embarrassing.

16. I would be prepared to tell a man if he were not making love to me the way I liked best (a) certainly; (b) only if I thought he could accept such a criticism; (c) never.

17. The ideal number of times to make love each week is (a) seven or more times; (b) three–four times; (c) once or twice.

18. In a new or casual sexual relationship, it is the man's duty to make sure that you are using a condom (a) the responsibility should be shared; (b) it is mostly the man's responsibility; (c) it is completely the man's responsibility.

19. Women have as much right to sexual satisfaction as men (a) yes; (b) probably, but their needs are different; (c) no.

20. I wish I could do something dramatic to change my sex life (a) yes; (b) yes, but not *too* dramatic! (c) no, I wouldn't like to.

This questionnaire is not based on strict scientific principles, but with the assistance of an advising psychiatrist I *have* prepared it with the intention of giving you a clear thumbnail sketch of how you feel about yourself sexually, and how far you might be prepared to go in order to refresh your love life.

If you scored more *a*'s than *b*'s or *c*'s, then you have already recognized the strength of your sexual needs, which are very powerful (but by no means abnormal!). Don't worry—you're not a nymphomaniac—nymphomania is actually a clinical condition that is extremely rare and is characterized by a chronic inability to achieve sexual satisfaction.

However, you do need arousing and satisfying love-making as often as possible, and you are prepared to admit it to yourself—and, given the chance, to any man who might come into your life. You are a prime candidate for improving your sex life very quickly and with spectacular results. You are expressive and outgoing and you are usually confident, but you do have doubts about yourself sexually and you are sometimes concerned that you are oversexed.

You may have recently experienced a disappointing marriage or sexual relationship but you strongly suspect that what went wrong was not your fault, and that you had every right to demand what you wanted (and what you didn't get.) In spite of your interest in sex and your need for regular sexual satisfaction, you are not very experienced. However, you are prepared to try almost anything for the thrill of it, because you recognize that, sensibly handled, and with all due precautions taken to protect you from pregnancy and sexually transmitted diseases, sex can give you and your partner huge emotional and physical pleasures. You know that when you find the right partner you will be prepared to give him everything and anything, and that your sexuality will blossom.

Eventually, you will form a long-lasting and very satisfying sexual relationship, and will experience sexual delights that seem "forbidden" to you now, but which will bring you excitement that up until now you have only fantasized about.

If you scored more *b*'s, then you are a giving and sexually aware person but you are still unsure about your sexual knowledge and how to deal with your own sexual needs, and you tend to rely on the guidance of your lovers when it comes to expressing yourself in bed.

Your early experiences of sex were not very satisfactory, and you have had at least one sexual experience in your teenage years or early twenties that could definitely be classed as traumatic. As a result, you have been deterred from committing yourself too much when it comes to lovemaking, and you have also been put off one or more sexual variations, such as oral or anal sex.

However, you are broadminded and emotionally well balanced, and if the right opportunity and the right partner present themselves, you will be willing to make an effort to overcome your inhibitions and try to enjoy those sexual variations that your previous experiences have spoiled for you.

You are naturally cautious, but once you are sure that your new partner will try his best to please and satisfy you, and that he will not try to bully you sexually or take you for granted, you are prepared to be deeply loyal and to give your relationship everything you've got.

There are some aspects of sex that worry you because you're not too sure about them, particularly aspects of male sexuality. How much sex does a man really need? How does he like you to caress his penis? If you say *no* to a man once he's aroused, will it do him any physical damage? Is there a time of the month when a man has a lower sperm count and is less likely to make you pregnant?

You're prepared to learn more about sex, however, given the right information and the right encouragement, and you're prepared to overcome your caution and your residual shyness if it really proves to pay dividends in terms of love and affection, and the kind of man who can satisfy you in bed.

If your score was predominantly *c*'s, then (through no fault of your own) you have clamped a lid over your own sexual desires. You have decided that sex is too risky, messy, dangerous, threatening, and disgusting, and that you would prefer not to have very much to do with it, except when absolutely necessary.

Although you may not have been a very highly sexed person to start with, your inhibited attitude toward sex has been developed almost entirely through clumsy, painful, and emotionally hurtful experiences. It's possible that you suffered some sexual abuse when you were very young. But it's more likely that your first sexual encounters were hostile and unpleasant and that you felt right from the very beginning that you were being sexually used, and that your partner or partners cared very little for what you felt or what you needed.

To protect yourself from further hurt and your sexuality from any further intrusion, you have kept yourself well away from the risk of falling in love, to the point where you have become sarcastic and flippant and hard shelled to any man who expresses an interest in you. Sometimes you wish that you didn't act that way. Sometimes you wish that you would bite your own tongue off. But keeping yourself to yourself, sexually, has become a habit that is very hard for you to shake.

You deny that you have sexual fantasies and a sexual appetite, but in fact yours are just as strong as that of any other woman. You have explicit pornographic fantasies, which you would never dream of revealing to anyone, but you also have sweeping romantic fantasies, too, like a one-woman production of *Gone with the Wind*.

One of the first things you have to overcome before you can find yourself an exciting and satisfying love life is your self-deprecating attitude toward your own body and the way you look. You take a great deal of care over your hair and grooming, and you almost always dress well, but you are still not convinced that you are really attractive to men. You are proud of your femininity and strongly interested in the advancement of women, but at the same time you have ambivalent feelings toward your own body.

You have a great deal to think about and a great many hang-ups to resolve before you can enter into a full and uninhibited sexual relationship, but the very fact that you are reading this book is a sign that you are more than willing to learn—even if you won't allow yourself to admit it. You have a strong and very sincere desire to find yourself an exciting and appreciative sex partner. If you are patient with yourself, and if you can learn to lower your guard with the men you meet, you will soon find that forming a good sexual relationship is neither as difficult nor as frightening as you keep imagining it to be.

The answers to most of the questions in this profile are self-evident, and you will be able to see for yourself what the ratio of *a*'s to *b*'s to *c*'s really indicates. If you have scored all *c*'s, it doesn't mean for a moment that you are sexually repressed, any more than scoring all *a*'s indicates that you are something of a sex maniac. The scores are intended to do nothing more than give you guidelines and suggestions, so that you can analyze more clearly some of the sexual problems that are worrying you, and some of the inhibitions that are holding you back.

It always helps to write down your feelings on paper. It gives you a clearer idea of what your inhibitions are—and of what your goals are, too.

Next, you should think about writing down your erotic fantasies, so that you can understand your own sexual tastes and how you can apply that knowledge to forming a new sexual relationship with a man.

Here's one girl who did, 26-year-old Velma, an unmarried redhead from Cleveland. "I had a fantasy that I was a white slave being sold in a slave market someplace in the Middle East. I was completely naked except for a silver collar around my neck, and silver shackles around my ankles. I was bought by this tall, handsome chieftain with a turban and a gold-embroidered bolero and a bare muscular chest, like those actors you see in those Sinbad movies. He dragged me into a tent in the desert and made me sit on a heap of cushions. Then he invited thirty or forty of his friends to watch me while I danced for them. I had to dance this incredibly lewd dance, caressing my breasts and licking my lips. I had to dance right up to these Arab men, and stand in front of them swaying my hips with my legs a little bit parted, so that they could give my cunt a quick lick. Then I had to lie back on the cushions, and open my legs up wide, and pull my cunt lips apart with my fingers, and slowly mastur-bate myself, thrusting my hand into my cunt, while they all sat around watching me.

"Then the handsome chieftain stood up and stripped off all of his clothes, and his cock was hard and enor-mous, the color of mahogany, and pulsing. He knelt between my legs, and pushed his cock up inside me, and all of his friends whistled and cheered. He fucked me, slow and beautiful, you could never imagine a man fucking you quite so slow and quite so beautiful, such a rhythm, and I could look down and see his mahogany-colored cock sliding in and out of my open cunt lips. I can still see it now, like a movie; or like I was really there.

"Then all of his friends stood up, and formed a circle all around us, and they all took out their cocks and slowly started to jack off, singing this Arabic chant while they did so. The chieftain had a climax, right inside me, I could feel my cunt filling up, and then all the other guys climaxed too, pulling themselves off, so that it was literally raining drops of warm sperm, all over me, all over my breasts and my stomach and my legs, and the chieftain massaged it all over my body, round and round, all over my breasts, and then slowly fucked me again, without hardly going soft in between.

"Afterwards I was chained up outside in the desert, like a dog, and any man who came past and wanted to jack off over my breasts or my face, or wanted me to suck his cock, I just had to do it. I was a complete slave."

The fascinating part about Velma's fantasy was that, in real life, she was very far from being "a complete slave." In fact, she was very sexually demanding—even domineering. But now let's see how she used her erotic fantasy to understand her sexuality—and to develop, as near as she knew how, her ideal sexual relationship.

FOUR

Single Sexual Fantasies

From a very early age, almost every woman has an idealized notion of the kind of man she would like to have as a lover—and, eventually perhaps, as a husband. As she grows older, her fantasy may become more pragmatic. She may gradually begin to understand, for instance, that handsome princes are in pretty short supply, or that there's only one Richard Gere and he's already far too old for her. She may also begin to recognize the value of other, less fantastic attributes, such as honesty and integrity and kindness.

Some women never quite manage to come to terms with the reality of men, which is that they're not always good looking or wealthy or hard working or sophisticated. Gina, 31, a homemaker from Tucson, Arizona, told me: "I despair of Marty. I always wanted a man to take me out to restaurants . . . a bronzed, handsome man in a white tuxedo. Well, Marty's handsome, and he's bronzed, and he even owns a white tuxedo. But when it comes to taking me out to restaurants, he's so unimaginative. He likes steak or chicken or ribs, and that's it. He knows two wines—white and red. Mostly, he prefers beer.

"I've tried to teach him some more sophistication when it comes to eating out, but he always says that food is food, and he knows what food he likes, so why should he try something that he knows that he's *not* going to like? I remember we went to a cocktail party once for some very good friends of ours, and he tried an oyster patty. He took one bite, and then he said, very loudly, 'Jesus, Gina, I think something's died in my muffin.' "

Gina loved Marty, and even after seven years of marriage she was very strongly attracted to him physically. But even in bed, his resistance to adventure occasionally made her despair. "He's a very tender lover, very gentle. But I see movies where the man tears off the woman's clothes and bends her over the back of the couch and has his way with her. Not violent, you know, but *raunchy*. And I see women with stockings and garter belts and high-heeled shoes on, in *bed* you know, screaming and bouncing around while their lover's socking it to them every which way. And I see movies where couples are having it out in the open air. And standing up in the shower stall. And almost every conceivable place and position you can think of.

"But Marty won't do that. I think he read a book when he was a boy that said a considerate man has to shower and trim his toenails and shave and brush his teeth and put on his nice clean pajamas. Then—and *only* then—is he fit to get into bed with his wife. He's very *clean*, I'll give him that much, and he makes love very tenderly—the way you'd imagine Robert Mitchum making love (although he probably doesn't), smooth and slow and almost asleep.

"But I do have fantasies about a sweaty, hairy-chested man breaking into the house, and dragging my clothes off, and forcing me down on the floor. He would kiss me with stale, garlicky breath, and then he would twist and bite my nipples. Then he would grab hold of my hair and push his huge piss-stinking cock into my mouth, right down my throat, so that I couldn't breathe anything but sweaty balls and ripe asshole.

"After he'd fucked me in the mouth as much as he wanted, he would turn me over on to my stomach and force his cock into my cunt. And he would grunt, and he would *grunt*, until I finally felt his cum burst out his cock.

"Afterward, he would turn me over again, and slap my face hard; and that would be the last I ever saw of him."

While Gina's fantasy may seem masochistic—the classic submissive fantasy of the rape victim—it was in fact quite the opposite. It was a strong, demanding fantasy—a fantasy that showed how urgent her need was for Marty to play his full masculine role in their sexual relationship. You should never think of your erotic fantasies as dirty daydreams to be ashamed of; neither should you think of them as evidence of sexual weakness or a perverted view of sex.

Your erotic fantasies are nothing more than conscious imaginary expressions of your sexual needs. Whether your needs are strong enough to want to play out your fantasies in real life has to be up to you to decide. Would you really get a kick out of being tied up? Would it really turn you on to meet your lover in a strange hotel, wearing nothing but high-heeled shoes and red PVC raincoat? Would you like to be fucked by two men at once? Or by a man and another girl? Would you like to pose nude in front of an audience?

These are questions that you can really only answer for yourself. But be warned: While you may have a strong and repeated fantasy of a particular sexual experience, the real experience may not be anything like you had always imagined it to be. A good case in point is Sylvia, a 27-year-old high-school teacher from Los Angeles who had fantasies for over seven years about being cornered in the school building and sexually attacked by senior boys.

"I suppose my subconscious was responding to the way in which they treated me during the school day. Six or seven of them were very handsome. They were also young, and fit, and cool. Whenever I walked past, one of them would clap his hands together and call out, 'Ow!' and all the rest of them would start baying like a pack of hounds.

"I had this repeated fantasy that I was locking up the school one night and I heard a noise, you know, like the scuffling of Nikes on a polished school floor. The next thing I knew, these double doors were thrown open and nine or ten boys rushed in and grabbed me. I screamed, but they forced a rag into my mouth. Then they carried me to the gym. I tried to kick and I tried to struggle, but there were too many of them—and, anyway, I was oddly aroused as well as frightened. It was the sexual fear of being hurt; the sexual fear of doing something dirty and forbidden; the sexual excitement of thinking that I had no control over the situation whatsoever.

"In a way, I suppose, that's a kind of masochism—a kind of bondage without ropes and handcuffs. It's also a way of thinking about sex without having any moral responsibility for what's happening in your mind—after all, you're only the victim, aren't you? Forget the fact that you invented everybody else in the fantasy. You're the innocent victim, kicking and struggling while those imaginary punks have their way with you. And how. I was never so comprehensively fucked as I was in fantasies.

"In the gym fantasy, they strapped me face upward on the vaulting horse, with my legs and arms wide apart. The leader leaned over me and grinned. He was ugly and unshaven, with a scarf around his head. He reminded me of one of the more delinquent boys in the sixth grade. In fact, it *was* him, in a way. He picked up a long thin-bladed knife and ran his thumb along the edge. It drew blood, and he pushed his thumb into my mouth and said, 'Suck it.' I said, 'What about

AIDS?' and he said, 'By the time we're through with you, sugar, AIDS will be the very least of your worries.'

"He stripped off his T-shirt and his jeans, and underneath his jeans he was wearing a tight black leather thong. His hard-on was so big that the head of his cock was rearing out of the top of his thong. It was deep purple, because the thong was binding it so tight, and there was clear juice dripping out of the opening, because he wanted to fuck me so much—me, his teacher, who spent the whole day telling him what to do.

"He climbed onto the vaulting horse, on top of me. He was so thin that I could see his ribs, but he was muscular, too. His body was covered in scars. I like men with scars: It proves they've suffered, and I think that's erotic. His armpits were hairy and there was hair on his chest.

"He pulled off his thong and then he was completely naked. His cock was standing out stiff. He leaned over me and licked my face all over, and then licked around my mouth, and then pushed his tongue into my mouth. Then he kissed my nipples, and bit them, and even *chewed* them, until I cried out in pain. Of course, when you fantasize about pain it isn't the same as real pain. It's just like an *idea* of being hurt.

"I have to confess that I do get excited when a man is dominant, and a little rough, and treats me like his whore. I don't know whether you would call that masochism or not. Personally, I think there's a little bit of the masochist in every woman's character, it's just part of her sexuality. But being a little bit masochistic isn't the same thing as being submissive, or weak, or allowing the man in your life to crush you completely. You get men who go to prostitutes, don't you, and have themselves tied up or whipped and stuff like that, but quite often those men are really powerful businessmen, guys who are in total control of everything they do.

"Anyway, this gym fantasy continued with two of the boys holding my pussy open and another one taking hold of the leader's cock and guiding it in between my legs. When I'm really involved in this fantasy, I can almost *feel* his cock sliding into me, as if it's actually happening. I don't know how I do that, maybe I just contract my pussy muscles or something. I don't use a vibrator or anything like that, no. But I open up my pussy with my fingers and close my eyes and I can almost *feel* that fat purple cock head sinking into me.

"He started to fuck me, and the others all clustered around me and shouted encouragement. They used all kinds of filthy language, all the disgusting things I hear boys saying around the school, and which I usually reprimand them for, or pretend that I haven't heard. Like 'Fuck her, fuck her, split that cunt," over and over. They chanted louder and louder, 'Fuck—her—fuck—her—' and I was begging them to stop, but the leader was pushing himself into me harder and harder, and even though I hated it, I loved it, too; it was turning me on so much. Suddenly I climaxed. I had an orgasm—even before he did.

"That turned the tables completely. He started to fuck me harder and harder, to prove that he could climax quickly, too. But I was in control now, not him, and he was the one who was panicking. He climaxed, and took out his cock, and sprayed his sperm everywhere, all over my stomach, all over the floor, and his friends shouted and clapped and whistled; but I knew then that *I* was the winner.

"He climbed off me, and looked hurt, like a bruised and beautiful fawn, with a lovely flat stomach and curved thighs. His cock was soft and shining, still swollen, and dripping with sperm.

"That was the end of *that* fantasy, more or less, although I have had similar fantasies, with a similar theme. I've thought about boys following me home after school, and catching me alone in a pedestrian tunnel, all wet and dark, and stripping off all of my clothes, and fucking me up against the wall, five or six of them, in silence, not one of them speaking, once. I've thought about boys breaking into my home at night, and gagging me, and pulling up my nightgown, and fucking me, one after the other. But even though you'd think these were masochistic fantasies, and maybe there *is* quite a lot of masochism in them, I always seem to get the upper hand. Usually because I like what they're doing to me . . . usually because I have an orgasm . . . even before they've started enjoying it themselves.

"Maybe the fact is that men may feel like dominating women, but they need women, too, and so women can give just as much or as little as they want."

Sylvia has a very sensible attitude toward her sexual fantasies. Her fantasies don't mean for a moment that she *really* wants to be raped by six or seven of the handsomest young men in her class. But they are an honest acknowledgement of the fact that she finds many of her senior pupils sexually attractive. In just the same way, many male teachers find themselves sexually aroused by the pubescent girls in their classes. It's a normal and understandable response. After all, the sexual age limits that society has drawn up are in reality quite artificial. They represent nothing more than our social consensus that young and innocent people should not be exploited by older people seeking sexual gratification.

Sylvia has never had an affair with any boy at the school where she teaches, nor would she consider it. But there is no school rule that says she can't fantasize, provided she keeps a sense of proportion and remembers at all times that she is a member of the school faculty, with all of the responsibilities toward her pupils that such a position of trust involves.

None of us need ever be ashamed of our fantasies, no matter how extreme they are. You may fantasize about cross-dressing or group sex or bondage or rape or orgies, but that doesn't mean for a moment that you are ever likely to take part in such activities, or that there is something "wrong" with you. Sexual fantasies are nothing more than a way of arousing yourself—a kind of mental masturbation. But even more than that, sexual fantasies are a very good way of discovering what turns you on and what *doesn't* turn you on. If you allow your mind to wander through all kinds of erotic imaginary sexual situations, it's surprising what you can discover about yourself.

Ellie, for example—a 27-year-old hair stylist from Indianapolis—has recurrent fantasies about competing to be Miss Nude America.

"It's the greatest turn-on. I imagine myself walking onto the stage, under the spotlights, wearing high heels and nothing else. My hair's all beautifully groomed, my makeup's perfect, my nails are perfect, my legs are waxed, my bikini area's waxed, I have a perfect all-over tan . . . and I stand on the stage stark naked in front of all of the cameras and all of the cheering crowds, and it's the greatest turn-on you can think of."

Would she actually do it, if she were chosen?

"No way . . . I'd be far too shy. I wouldn't appear naked in front of anybody else except my husband. But my fantasy gave me the idea of posing for *him*—you know, opening the door for him when he comes home, completely naked, spending the morning naked, making his breakfast naked. He loves it, he really thinks it's a turn-on, and it gives *me* a chance to preen myself, too. I guess you could say that I've always been vain—you know, fussy with my grooming, and I like to show myself off to him."

Jane, 33, a realtor from Minneapolis, had fantasies about meeting a complete stranger and having sex with

him, without a word being exchanged between them—
rather like the Marlon Brando/Maria Schneider movie
Last Tango in Paris. She told her 35-year-old lover Paul
about them and he suggested that he visit some of the
houses where she was holding open days and make
love to her.

"It was such an incredible success. Paul really entered into the spirit of it, and wore different disguises
and different clothes. Sometimes we laughed ourselves
silly, but then he would lock the front door and take
me upstairs, into somebody else's bedroom, and take
off my clothes and fuck me without a single word.
Sometimes there would be prospective buyers, banging
on the door to view the house. But he would keep on
fucking me, totally silent. I can't explain how spooky
and scary and erotic it was."

Michelle, a 23-year-old computer programmer, had
fantasies about being tied up to the bed and blind-
folded, while two or even three men "had their way"
with her. "I imagined them touching my lips with their
cocks, one at a time, or all together, and I wouldn't
know which cock belonged to which man . . . and then
one of them would start licking me between my legs,
and another would massage my breasts with his cock,
and another one would be running his fingers all over
me. And I would never know who they were, or how
many there were, or whether they were handsome or
ugly or black or white. I had another fantasy about two
men forcing their cocks into my mouth, side by side,
so that I was practically gagging, but all the same I
wanted them both, I *wanted* them to choke me, almost,
they were so stiff and salty and rubbery. Then I tugged
off my blindfold and discovered that one cock was
black and the other cock was white, and for some reason that *really* made me flip." (Michelle herself is
black.)

Michelle used her fantasies to enliven her own sex

life by asking her boyfriend to blindfold her and then "do to me whatever it entered his head to do to me." One of the results was 20 minutes of "total delight" in which her boyfriend massaged her breasts and stimulated her clitoris and her vagina with his fingers and gave her "two orgasms . . . three . . . four . . . I can scarcely recall. It was just one orgasm after another. He only stopped when I couldn't stand it anymore, and started to scream!"

But it isn't always necessary or desirable to act out your fantasies for real. You might have a very exciting fantasy about taking a .38 revolver into work and blowing your boss's head off. Of course, you can get pleasure from such a fantasy, and it can tell you a lot about your day-to-day relationship with your boss. But it certainly wouldn't further your career or improve your life in any way at all. It's the same with erotic fantasies. The images in your mind may arouse you tremendously. But you have to use some judgment when it comes to turning those images into reality. Your partner may find some of your sexual desires extreme or shocking, and you yourself may very well find that what turns you on as a fantasy a very big turn-off when you try to do it for real.

A case in point is Nan, 32, a homemaker from Seattle: "For years I had fantasies about a man putting me over his knee and spanking me with a hairbrush. I always imagined it would be sharp and tingly and very, very sexy. I used to think about a man spanking me and masturbate. I rubbed my thighs and my bottom with my hairbrush, or brushed my pubic hair very fiercely, and sometimes I slid the handle up inside my vagina. I told myself that I was a naughty girl, and that I deserved to be spanked. I could bring myself to an orgasm, just by thinking about it.

"About three years ago, I met a man through a dating agency and we hit it off immediately. We had everything in common—our taste in music, our taste in humor, our taste in food. We both enjoyed sailing and horseback riding. We loved Chinese restaurants. His name was Max and he was tall and gray haired and athletic. Maybe he wasn't as handsome as I could have wished, but he was very warm and physical, very touchy-feely.

"We started a sexual affair, and it was good, but it never seemed to have any *fire*, do you know what I mean? It was all too polite, all too caring. Max was too much of a gentleman. One day he took me out for lunch and he'd bought this really expensive yachting blazer. Afterward, he took me back to his apartment, the way he always did, so that we could go to bed. I was undressing, and he was undressing, but instead of kissing me and nuzzling my neck and all of that smoochy stuff, he was hanging up his new blazer, and brushing it, and making sure all of the buttons were shiny. I said, 'You care more about that expletive deleted blazer than you do about me!' He said, 'I do not!' and I said, 'Do too!' and to prove it I tipped a whole glass of red wine all over it.

"Max was furious. So I challenged him. I said, 'If you're so furious, why don't you spank me?' And, by God, he did. He took hold of me and he put me over his knee and he dragged down my panties and he spanked me. And it *hurt*. I can't tell you how much it hurt. You can tell all of those women who have ever fantasized about being spanked that it *hurts*. You should have seen my bottom afterwards. It was bright red and covered in handprints.

"We made love that afternoon, and it *was* more exciting . . . just for that one afternoon, anyway. But it was only exciting because something violent had happened between us, and we were making up. Afterward, as we lay in bed together and the room was growing darker, I knew for sure that our relationship was finished. It's very exciting to have fantasies about spanking and whipping and suchlike in your head, but if you're tempted to act them out for real, then I think you need to take a close look at what's wrong with your relationship, don't you agree? You shouldn't need to hurt your partner to get turned on, or to think that you have to be hurt in return."

Of course, Nan raised a very complex question about pain and pleasure. There are many people who *do* like some ingredient of pain or discipline in their sexual relationships, and there are some people who are unable to reach a climax without it.

Sylvia, the schoolteacher, rightly mentioned that there are many men in responsible positions of authority who seek the services of dominant prostitutes. Although they are totally in charge of their careers, they can only find sexual satisfaction if they are being tied up or humiliated or treated like helpless children.

Some years ago, I was friendly with Monique von Cleef, the notorious Dutch dominatrix, and she showed me around her "torture chamber" in the Hague, where judges, police chiefs and leading businessmen would regularly visit her and pay generously for sexual humiliation. She would hang them up by their heels from the ceiling and administer huge warm-water enemas which they were forbidden to expel. She would make them sit on a milking stool with a seat that featured a nine-inch wooden dildo in the middle and tell her nursery stories. She would mask them in leather and buckle "dog's-muzzles" full of inward-pointing spikes over their penises.

Obviously, the services that Monique was providing were quite extreme. But we shouldn't miss the point here. Whether we try to act them out or not, our erotic fantasies are an expression of the way we feel about ourselves and about our role in life, and a vivid indication of what we are looking for in a sexual relationship.

From her sexual fantasies, any single woman can quite clearly gauge the level of her sexual self-confidence—and prepare a profile of the kind of man who would be most likely to give her the sexual satisfaction that she is looking for.

This quiz is designed to help you to assess your sexual needs. Ask yourself each question as truthfully and as frankly as you can, and then write your answers in a list on a separate sheet of paper. You may be surprised by the profile of your sexual personality that emerges.

You may also be surprised how sexually adventurous you are prepared to be.

1. *What is the most significant character of your sexual fantasies?* (a) One-to-one sex with a man with whom you're already intimate; (b) One-to-one sex with a man you know but with whom you are not yet intimate; (c) One-to-one sex with a completely imaginary man; (d) One-to-one sex with a famous movie or singing star or similar; (e) Sex with two–three men; (f) Sex with countless numbers of men.

2. *When you fantasize about sex, is it:* (a) In private; (b) In front of other people; (c) In front of crowds of spectators.

3. *In your sexual fantasies, are you:* (a) Yourself, as you are; (b) Yourself, with cosmetic alterations; (c) Somebody else altogether; (d) A spectator, and not a participant.

4. *In sexual fantasies, are you usually:* (a) Dressed in high fashion; (b) Dressed in short skirts and revealing tops; (c) Dressed in erotic underwear—stockings and garter belts; (d) Dressed in romantic silk robes; (e) Naked.

5. *Are the men in your sexual fantasies:* (a) Submissive; (b) Kind and gentle; (c) Romantic and

courteous; (d) Passionate and wilful; (e) Ragingly lustful; (f) Violent and rapacious.

6. *Are the men in your sexual fantasies:* (a) Clean and well groomed; (b) dirty and rough.

7. *By your real-life standards, is the sex in your fantasies:* (a) Ordinary; (b) Unusual; (c) Perverted.

8. *What is the dominant sexual theme in your fantasies?* (a) One-to-one intercourse; (b) Oral sex (you giving it to him); (c) Oral sex (him giving it to you); (d) Group sex (several men, one woman); (e) Group sex (several women, one man); (f) Bondage (you tied up); (g) Bondage (him tied up); (h) Leather or rubber or similar fetishistic clothing; (i) Tattooing, or any kind of piercing (nipples, foreskins, vaginal lips); (j) Anal sex; (k) Fisting—the insertion of the whole hand into vagina or anus; (l) Wet sex—erotic play with urine; (m) Other.

9. *How often do you think about your favorite sexual fantasy?* (a) Every day; (b) Once or twice a week; (c) Once or twice or month; (d) Once or twice a year.

10. *Would you tell your lover about your favorite sexual fantasy?* (a) Of course; (b) It would depend on what kind of lover he was; (c) I might consider it; (d) Never.

11. *Would you like to act out your sexual fantasy for real?* (a) Yes, in every detail; (b) Only part of it; (c) No.

At the end of your list, write down one sexual fantasy which you have never divulged to anybody, and see what you think about it when you look at it in the bold, honest light of day.

Erotic fantasies can help us to define what kind of sexual people we are. From the content of our fantasies, we can quickly and clearly decide whether we're mostly dominant or mostly submissive, or whether we have a particular erotic taste that excites us more than any other.

For a single woman, understanding her erotic fantasies is extremely important. They can help her to shape her attitude toward the men she meets, and know what she wants from them sexually. They can help her to refine her sexual criteria. If a woman is always sexually dominant in her fantasies—if she is strongly aroused by the thought of treating men as sexual slaves—then she may be well advised to think twice about forming a relationship with a man who is equally dominant. The result could be more catastrophic than just a clash of personalities. A man who enjoys being sexually dominant could well be infuriated and frustrated by a woman who likes to take charge in the bedroom.

Mamie, a 27-year-old interior decorator from Chicago, had a favorite fantasy of treating men like slaves.

"My father was a very strong personality, very dominant. I think I inherited my personality from him. Apart from that, I'm tall, I'm brunette, I'm up-front, I never mince my words. I think I'm attractive, too, although it embarrasses me to say so. Years and years ago when I was a girl I read a book that my father had left lying around called *Fort Frederick,* which was about a man who is treated as a slave by the woman of the house. The idea of that fascinated me and really turned me on. You know those times when you're going through puberty and you have such sexy feelings sometimes you feel as if you're going to fizz, like a shook-up bottle of soda? Well, that's how I used to feel when I thought about having a man for a slave. He would be very good looking and sulky and dark haired and muscular. He would have to be naked all of the time, except when he was cooking or dusting or serving me meals, when he would have to wear a white frilly apron. If I wanted to reach under his apron and fondle his cock and his balls, he would have to let me. He would have to let me do whatever I wanted. He would have to bathe me, and wash me in the shower, and paint my fingernails and toenails. If I wanted to lie in bed all morning reading magazines and eating chocolates while he licked my cunt, he would have to do it. I could just imagine it, lying back in this beautiful four-poster bed with the sun streaming through the window, eating a whole boxful of Stouffer's pecan creams, naked except for a silky negligée, my legs wide apart, while this gorgeous handsome hunk of a man played his tongue all over my clitoris, and massaged his whole face into my slippery-wet cunt. If I wanted him to fuck me in the wee small hours of the night, he would have to do it. If I wanted him to stand beside my chair so that I could suck his cock whenever it took my fancy, he would have to do it. It was my absolute favorite fantasy, and it kind of took on a life of its own. I always had this gorgeous man in the back of my mind. He didn't even have a name, but he always did what I wanted, and he never argued, and he was always completely submissive. Sometimes I would have fantasies about him that were only mildly sexual . . . like, he had to serve me breakfast, and he would be naked, and I would take a handful of scrambled eggs off my plate and massage his balls and his cock with them, and squidge them into his pubic hair. Then other times the fantasies would be pretty extreme . . . like, I would have to punish him by strapping him with leather anklets to the head of his bed, and whip his cock with a little stinging leather whip. He would scream out, but he would climax, too, and I would be whipping sperm everywhere, all around the room. Sometimes I would be real severe, and he would have to do *everything* for me. After I'd been to the bathroom, I would bend over, and he would have to lick me totally clean, really taking his time, really probing, and his face would be smothered in shit. Then he would have to run my bath for me and pamper me with perfume powder and carry me to bed."

Although I have necessarily abridged it for the purposes of this book, it took Mamie a long time to confess to the whole of this fantasy. But, having done so, she realized that it was a very vivid dramatization of her feelings about men. She may have fantasized so graphically about having a male sex slave because she had inherited her father's dominant personality. However, his dominant personality may also have led her to yearn for a man who was totally submissive, totally benign, and who would give her all the comfort and sexual pleasure she wanted without expecting anything in return.

I asked Mamie whether her father had ever abused her in any way, but she had no memory of it, except to say that he had continued to walk into the bathroom unannounced for two or three years after she had reached puberty, which had deeply embarrassed her.

Because she was so attractive, Mamie had very little trouble attracting men. But her problem was that she was *so* attractive that she always ended up with the most dominant men (because, rather like lions, they had "seen off" all the meeker contenders.)

"In my early twenties, I had three disastrous relationships with very strong, good-looking men. All of them had a great deal in common with my father. They were self-confident, they knew what they wanted out of life. Also, they treated me like some kind of pet. I hated all three of those relationships. Every one of them ended in a hideous argument. I spent over a year on my own, keeping away from men, keeping away from any kind of sexual relationship. Then a friend suggested I should place a personal ad. She said that it had taken some time, but it had really worked for her. I couldn't believe that she had found the man she was going to marry from a personal ad! I mean, I had talked to the guy dozens of times and I never would have guessed that she had found him through a magazine!

"She gave me a whole lot of advice about writing a personal ad, and told me that it was important to think about my sexual fantasies. She said: 'Dream your dream. You may find somebody, you may not. But at least you know what you're going for.'

"So that's what I did. And that's how I met Jim. Well, not instantly—it took six or seven bum dates first! Jim and I aren't engaged to be married yet, or anything like that, but the chances are that we will be. He's quiet, he's reserved, he loves me—and I love him. He's strong, but he allows me to be strong, too, and doesn't feel embarrassed about it. He's never upset if I want to sit on top of him when we're making love, and he never feels threatened if I make the first move. I don't want to act out the whole of my fantasy with him. For instance, I wouldn't want him to do all the housework and wear an apron. But sometimes I ask him not to dress in the morning, and to walk around naked, and I love that, I really do. It excites me! I have a totally naked man in my apartment, and I can do anything with him!"

Mamie recognized that her fantasies held the key to her sexual personality. As I have said many times before, fantasies are only figments of our erotic imaginations. They're not real—they're simply the way we use our minds to excite ourselves sexually. We have no need to be ashamed of them, no matter how "perverted" or "kinky" they may seem to be—and, of course, they often seem "perverted" and "kinky" when we think about them later, in the cold light of day when we're no longer sexually aroused.

For a single woman to have an erotic fantasy is no worse than having a fantasy about being rich or famous or stunningly beautiful. Perhaps the only difference is that she can learn something really practical from her erotic fantasies, and put that knowledge to work to change her life. Because whatever erotic fantasy a single woman may have, the chances are that there is a man out there, somewhere in this wide world, who is more than willing to fulfill it for her.

As Mamie finally admitted, "I had some bathroom fantasies that kind of made me blush to talk about them. Jim and I have never done anything so extreme as my fantasies. But one evening before my shower he came into the bathroom when I was sitting naked on the john, and he knelt down beside me and he kissed me so deep and so beautiful he made me shudder. And I was pissing at the time, but he reached down with his hand between my legs and he tickled my clitoris and slid his finger up inside my cunt, even though I was gushing piss into his hand. It was then I knew that he would do anything for me, just like the man in my fantasy."

You don't have to act out your fantasies in order for them to help you to improve your sex life. You don't even have to tell anybody else what they are. And you should never be ashamed of them. They may be totally outrageous, totally beyond the bounds of "good taste." But they don't affect your niceness, they don't affect your relationships with your friends or family. They're simply an imaginative manifestation of the passions and desires that *everybody* has within them.

I talked to a handsome, self-confident mother of five children in Milwaukee, who told me that she had always fantasized about crawling under a table at an expensive restaurant, opening the fly of a completely unsuspecting male diner "and sucking his cock until the tears came to his eyes." She had never done it for real. She had no intention *ever* of doing it for real. But it was a teasing, tantalizing, and erotic idea, and it very pleasantly turned her on, and there is no harm in that whatsoever. Apart from that, you should have tasted her blueberry muffins—anybody who bakes blueberry muffins like that can't be all kinky!

Before we go on to the physical and emotional tensions of being single, let's just take a look at some of the reasons why single women have stayed single.

The Women Who Expected Too Much

Jane, 35, a waitress from Pittsburgh: "I always had a dream of marrying a man who looked like John Travolta. Funny, handsome, caring, natural, a terrific dancer. A little bit goofy, too. I had two offers of marriage—one from Sal, who ran an auto-rental concession, handsome but no sense of humor. Then Jeff, who did something mysterious in travel insurance. He was funny, but he was awkward, too. He used to blush a whole lot. I don't know, he just didn't seem coordinated. He was very gentle and romantic when he made love to me. He used to make me feel good. But, I don't know. I always dreamed of something better. I go out on dates, sure. Sometimes, if I like a man a lot, I go to bed with him. But most of the time I go home and watch TV. My favorite is *Studs*."

The Women Who Expected Too Little

Jerri-Lee, 40, from Houston: "I was brought up in a family of seven girls where none of us were taught to expect anything but the same life that my momma had lived. My momma didn't live a life of drudgery but she was expected to know her place in life, which was cooking and cleaning and taking care of us kids. When I was about 21 I went to a barbecue with some friends of mine on Galveston Island and I was cornered by a real cute boy who never left me alone all evening. I gave him my address and the next day he came to call for me. He was driving a new white Mustang convertible! It turned out that he was the son of this top aerospace executive. He treated me like a princess. He took me dancing. He took me back to his own apartment and he made love to me. There was a mirror on the ceiling, right over the bed and I watched him making love to me. He had a beautiful back, I'll never forget looking up at him and seeing that beautiful back, and that tight bare bottom, and my own face, looking back at me. He took me out three or four times, and every single time we made love, and it was beautiful, and I loved it. Once he took me down by the bayou, and I knelt on the backseat, with my frock over my head and my panties round my knees, and he pushed himself into me, and pushed, and pushed, and it felt so beautiful I was crying, and there were my tears on that shiny white leather upholstery and I knew this wasn't for me. I wasn't good enough for this. Maybe I was scared that it was all a dream, and that I was going to wake up. Maybe I knew that he would have to hurt me, one day. Maybe I wanted to feel that I had some say over how our relationship went—not just him making all of the decisions, every time, and paying for everything—and paying for me, when it came down to it. I broke it off before *he* could break it off, to save myself the pain of it . . . although sometimes I wonder if he would've."

The Women Who Were Afraid of Committing Themselves

Kathleen, 32, a photographer from Seattle: "I'm a woman of powerful sexuality and I love men. In the whole of my lifetime I've had eight or nine love affairs, and only one of those affairs hasn't been sexual. I love touching men, I love photographing men. I have a book—as yet unpublished—which is nothing more than black-and-white photographs of men's penises, some resting, some half-erect, some fully erect. I adore fully-erect penises. I used to suck some of my models' penises to make them stiff, and whole dreamy hours would go by, while I sucked, and sucked. I would love to wake up every morning next to a man. But for some reason I've always been terrified of what might happen to me if I open my life to a man. I think he would probably trample all over my personality and leave me with nothing. I don't think that girls are brought up to understand men or that boys are brought up to understand women. I'm not sure. I'm terrified of giving myself away, and then finding that I can't get myself back again."

The Women Who Were Afraid of Sexually "Letting Go"

Iris, 23, a grade-school teacher from St. Louis: "My mother didn't tell me anything about sex except that men wanted it from you and it hurt. The stories they told at school didn't make it sound any better. I always had this very negative view of sex. It seemed like sex was something that other people did, and I didn't want to have any part of it. I had a bad experience at high school when a boy tried to rape me. Well, he didn't exactly try to rape me, but he kept trying to kiss me and touch my breasts and in the end I had to scream and push him off. After that I was known as 'Iceblock Iris', which didn't help my attitude toward sex. I've had one lesbian relationship even though I know that I'm not a lesbian. I met a girl called Carole when I was training to be a teacher and I suppose we were both lonesome. We slept together about six or seven times and she liked to caress my breasts and play with my clitoris and give me vaginal kisses. I would be lying if I said that I didn't enjoy sex with Carole, for as long as it lasted. She reassured me, gave me confidence. She made me feel that I was sexually attractive. The trouble was, I couldn't give her the same sexual stimulation in return. She would go down on me, and position her vagina right in front of my face, and open it wide with her fingers, trying to coax me into kissing her and licking her. She was beautiful; she didn't disgust me or anything. But I just couldn't do it. That made her angry after a while, and I'm not really surprised. I couldn't expect her to make me feel better without doing anything to make *her* feel better in return. We stopped sleeping together after about three months. Next I had a relationship with a boy called Terry who was very kind and understanding, but when he wanted more than just friendship, when he kissed me and tried to touch my breasts, I had to tell him that it was over. I'm *terrified* of sex. I don't know why. I think about it all the time. I feel so isolated. I feel as if I'm going to spend the rest of my life totally alone, without love or affection."

The Women Who Were Divorced or Separated

Moira, 36, from Newark, New Jersey: "I was married to Ted for over nine years, and I thought we had a wonderful marriage. I have two children from that marriage, a boy and a girl, six and four. When my marriage broke up, it came like a bolt from the blue. I know that our sex life hadn't been very passionate over the last two years of our marriage, but I put that down to the fact that I was raising two young children and holding down a part-time job and Ted was working all of the hours that God gave him. I thought we were building toward a happy and secure future. Instead, Ted suddenly announced that he was in love with another woman, and within a week he had left me. It knocked all of the confidence out of me. In the five minutes that it had taken Ted to tell me our marriage was over, my sexual self-esteem was totally destroyed. But of course that was only the tip of the iceberg. I picked myself up and dusted myself off, sure. I told myself that at the age of 35 I was still young and attractive. I almost believed myself. The trouble was, I was faced with the problem of finding myself a man who agreed with me. I felt like I'd contracted some kind of terrible social disease. All of my friends avoided me. I was scarcely ever invited to parties or dinners any more. Whenever I *was* invited, it was usually to find that I was being paired off with some hideous guy about twice my age with bad teeth and a toupee. Although our sex life hadn't been too good, I became sexually desperate. There was one evening when I seriously thought about becoming a prostitute or working in a massage parlor, just to feel a man's arms around me, just to feel a man's hard penis inside me. I miss the smell of a man, I miss the warmth of a man, I can't even describe to you how much. Do you know what I was thinking last week, when I was lying in bed? I never used to enjoy oral sex very much, because Ted liked to come in my mouth. I thought: I may never taste a man's sperm, ever again, in the whole of my life. I burst into tears. I used to have divorced and separated friends, and I used to envy them all of that free time. I used to say, I'd give anything just to be able to get up and go out whenever I felt like it, to wash my hair whenever I felt like, to eat tuna fish out of the can in front of the television with curlers in my hair. I can't tell you how much I regret saying those words today. I'd trade all of my so-called freedom right now, right this minute, for one loving kiss."

You'll be pleased to know that Moira did find herself a new partner, through a personal ad in a statewide magazine. She is now happily remarried and "very fulfilled, in every way."

Many single women find that they are able to cope with their sexual frustrations reasonably well. Claudia, a 25-year-old journalist, told me that "in between boyfriends, I divert all of my sexual energy into writing. I've produced some of my very best articles at times when I've been celibate."

Other single women are capable of remaining celibate for very long periods of time without feeling sexually frustrated. Naomi, 37, who works in a health-food store in San Francisco, said, "I enjoy the company of men, but I'm always happier when I'm not sexually involved. I feel more intensely *myself*, if you understand what I mean. I feel purer and simpler and I find myself much calmer and much more capable. Whenever I'm tangled up in a sexual relationship, I always experience terrible highs and lows—up one minute, down the next, not only emotionally but physically, too. Sex has made me happier than anything I know. It's also made me more depressed than anything I know. At the moment I've chosen the quiet, even path."

What can women do to satisfy themselves sexually when they're between lovers, or if they've chosen to be single, yet still feel strong sexual urges?

There was a time not too long ago when female masturbation was a taboo subject, but these days, fortunately, it is recognized as a perfectly healthy and sensible option for a woman with a sexual appetite but no lover to indulge it.

Let's take a look at some of the tried-and-tested ways of arousing yourself sexually, and some startling new ways, too.

FIVE

The Singular Act of Self-Stimulation

It wasn't long ago that women's magazines were far more likely to feature new ideas for macramé than masturbation—but these days, it's the other way around. We have come to accept and understand that there is nothing harmful or degrading about seeking sexual pleasure from stimulating our own minds and our own bodies.

In fact, masturbation can do a great deal to keep a single woman sane and happy and free from physical tensions. Of course, masturbation will never be a substitute for sexual intercourse. If you think of it as such, you will never be able to see it for what it is—a recreational activity that can bring you moments of intense pleasure, and which can help to relieve the stressful feelings of sexual frustration.

Kate, 24, a medical student from Boston, told me: "I never masturbated in early adolescence. It's hard to remember, but I don't think I even *knew* about masturbation. But when I was 15, I spent the summer with my cousins in San Diego, and I had to share a bedroom with Chrissie, who was a year older than me.

"When it came to bedtime, we talked for a while—I don't know, about our favorite rock stars and stuff like that. Then we switched off the light and *I* went to sleep. But Chrissie obviously didn't, because about quarter of 12 I heard these *noises* coming from her bed. She was groaning and gasping, and making all these peculiar panting sounds. I was terrified! I thought she was having a fit or something, or choking. I switched on the light and went around to her bed and said, 'Chrissie, are you all *right*?' and she looked up at me and said, 'Of course I'm all right, I'm diddling myself.'

"I didn't even know what she meant. I mean, I kind of *guessed* what she meant, but I had never heard anybody talking about it so openly before.

"She said, 'Don't you diddle?' And I said, 'No. I don't even know what diddling *is*.' But Chrissie said, 'All the girls do it. If you don't have a man, what else are you supposed to do?'

"I'd had plenty of sexy dreams and sexy fantasies. I mean, I'd thought about boyfriends and being married, and there was one boy at school called Clyde who used to wear these really tight swimshorts, and you could see practically every detail of his penis and everything.

"But my mom never told me much about sex. I asked her once about babies, and all she said was 'All in good time.' That was all I got from her, 'All in good time.' Only the 'good time' never seemed to come. Maybe she was embarrassed, I don't know. But I didn't know anything about masturbation until Chrissie showed me, and when she *did* show me, I could hardly believe that anything that felt so good could be so wrong.

"I said to Chrissie, 'What do you do?' And she said, 'You really don't know?'

"She threw back her bedcovers. She was wearing a stripy nightshirt, but she had pulled it way up above her waist. She was hot and her skin was shining with perspiration. She had been lying on her side but she turned onto her back and opened her legs. She was plump, but she had a very good figure. Big breasts, you know, and all the boys liked her.

"She didn't have any pubic hair at all. Her cunt was completely bare. I was really surprised because she was older than me. I was so naive I thought that she simply hadn't grown any yet! But she didn't say anything about it, and so I didn't. And after all, I was only 15, and some of my friends still hadn't grown much hair. She lay back and she said, 'Look, this is how you do it.'

"She opened her cunt lips very slightly with the fingers of her left hand, and then she placed the middle finger of her right hand on her clitoris. I was fascinated. I had seen girls naked before. I'd seen them in the shower, and in the locker room. But I had never been able to sit so close to a girl and actually watch her playing with her cunt, the way that Chrissie was.

"Her cunt lips were very pale pink, and they were shining with juice. I couldn't believe how wet she was. Her cunt itself was a little way open, so that I could see right up inside her, and she was so wet that the juice was dripping out of her cunt and down between the cheeks of her bottom. I think what excited me more than anything else was the fact that she wasn't at all embarrassed about what she was doing, and that it actually turned her on, displaying herself so openly.

"She started to flick her clitoris with her middle finger, so quickly that I could hardly see it. She said she liked it very fast and very, very light—so light that she could scarcely feel it, so that she kept on wanting more, and more, and more, but wouldn't let herself have it.

"She said, 'Wanting it, and being able to give it yourself, but never quite allowing yourself to have it—that's the secret.'

"When I watched her, I think I understood what she meant. She kept flicking her clitoris with her finger until I could see that her clitoris was rising and stiffening, it was hard and pink and triangular, and it really stuck out. But she didn't flick it any harder, she kept up that quick, light caress. She reached underneath her bottom with her left hand, and started to stroke her asshole. But it was only the lightest of touches, the tip of her fingernail circling her asshole. I could actually see her asshole *twitching*, as if she wanted nothing more in the world than to push her finger up into it, but she didn't. She just kept on diddling herself, faster and faster, light as a feather.

"She started to pant. She had a red flush, all across her chest. She opened her legs really wide, and she began to pull open the lips of her cunt, and slide her fingers inside, faster and faster, until her cunt and her fingers were all slippery with juice. I thought that she had completely forgotten about me, but she hadn't. She suddenly said, 'Kate . . . watch . . .' and she had an orgasm, right in front of me, clutching my hand, shaking, shuddering.

"I had started off by being shocked. But by the time Chrissie climaxed, I wasn't shocked any more, I was too excited. I suddenly thought: 'This is something that I can do, too, and it's obviously harmless, because Chrissie does it, and Chrissie is such a health-freak.'

"Chrissie said, 'Here . . .' and took hold of my hand, and tried to pull it down between her legs. I resisted, but then she said, 'It's okay . . . I just want to show you what it's like.' I touched her cunt, and it was like warm silk, only it was slippery, too. Then I slid one finger up inside her, and she was so wet and hot that I could hardly believe it. I'd never even done that to myself, let alone somebody else!

" 'Here . . .' she said, 'here,' and turned herself over, and stuck her bottom in the air. She took hold of my hand and guided my middle finger into her cunt, and my index finger toward her asshole. She had a beautiful pink asshole, and she kept on saying, 'Go on . . . go on . . . do what you want.' And in the end I slid my finger into her asshole, right up to the knuckle, and rubbed my two fingers together, the finger in her cunt and the finger in her asshole, rubbed them around and around, while Chrissie lay with her face buried in the pillow and just kept on saying, 'Oh . . . oh . . . oh . . .'

"It took her a long time to climax but I was wishing that she could hold off forever. To me, there was something so sexy about churning my fingers around and around inside another girl's bottom that I *never* wanted to stop. When she did finally climax, she reached around behind her and snatched my wrist and forced my fingers even more deep inside her. She screamed out, 'Hurt me!' although she denied later that she had ever said anything like that.

"That was how I learned to masturbate. I'm very much older now, and I've been through two serious sexual relationships with men (neither of which, unfortunately, turned out good). I'm not a lesbian, even though I respect lesbians' choice to have sex with whoever they want. I'm not a nymphomaniac or a pervert or any of those things. I'm simply a woman who spends a whole lot of nights on her own and gets pleasure and satisfaction out of diddling herself, the same way that Chrissie did . . . quick and light, holding back on myself, waiting, teasing, the very same thing.

"I don't like anal penetration . . . I've never taken to it. But I do get turned on by moistening my finger with a little Oil of Olay and circling it around and around my asshole while I masturbate. I must have the tenderest, most youthful-looking asshole ever!"

Until comparatively recently, masturbation (both male and female) was regarded not only as immoral, but physically and mentally harmful. I have an extraordinary collection of Edwardian engravings that depict girls who were driven to depression, madness, or even suicide by committing "the secret vice." Handbooks that were supposed to give young girls "the facts of life" sternly warned that self-stimulation would lead to blindness, deformity, sterility, frigidity, and feebleness of mind. In some extreme cases, excessive diddling could actually kill you.

> "Oh, sisters!" begged Mrs. Emma F. Angell Drake, M.D. "Let me beseech you, do not barter your birthright, your health, youth and beauty, for such a moldy mess of pottage, for depend upon it, death lurks beneath, and will spring out at you before your realize it!"

So fierce was the religious and social condemnation of masturbation that the term "self-abuse" can still be heard occasionally, even today—and I still receive letters from girls who are worried that masturbation might somehow affect their sexual responses or make it impossible for them to achieve orgasm "the normal way, with a man."

It's perfectly usual for young girls to feel furtive and ashamed when they first start masturbating in adolescence. This is sex! This must be dirty! Donna, now 32, a divorcee from Galveston, Texas, told me: "When I was 14, I prayed to God every single day to stop me from masturbating. I used to think that it showed on my face, that every single zit was caused by stroking myself. I used to feel really tired sometimes, and I was sure that my strength was being sapped by masturbating. But I couldn't stop it, I couldn't stop myself. I used to go to bed and lie there and start thinking about Mr. Heidelman, my art teacher, and the next thing I knew I was stroking myself again. I used to have an orgasm, and then pray for forgiveness. I guess I was like St. Augustine, 'Oh Lord, make me perfect, but not yet.' "

Even the most well-informed and well-adjusted girls feel confused and embarrassed during adolescence. That makes it doubly difficult for them to discuss the subject of masturbation with their mothers or teachers or anybody who could categorically reassure them that masturbation isn't at all harmful.

Masturbation is enjoyable, relaxing, and a useful aid to relieving every kind of stress. At worst, it's fun. At best, it can be a very effective way to achieve sexual self-understanding, both physically and emotionally.

Regrettably, even when a girl *does* pluck up the courage to ask about masturbation, there are still plenty of parents and doctors and youth counselors who believe that sexual self-stimulation is sinful and disgusting. And if a girl gets a strongly negative response to her need for information about masturbation when she's in adolescence, her feeling of shame may linger well into her twenties and thirties and even beyond, inhibiting her from enjoying masturbation at times when she most needs it.

Although surveys have indicated that well over three-quarters of all women in the United States admit to having masturbated regularly, most of the women to whom I talked in the preparation of this book were very reluctant at first to admit that one of those women might have been *them*.

I think Margaret, a 24-year-old hair stylist from Chicago, summed up the most succinctly: "If you admit that you masturbate, that means one of only two things. Either you don't have a man who satisfies you in bed, or you don't have a man at all. And what woman's going to admit to that?"

So, masturbation is widely associated with sexual and social failure, and that's why we don't like to say that we do it. But the extraordinary thing is that literally millions and millions of men and women masturbate with astonishing frequency, as the huge annual sales of masturbatory aids bear witness.

We spend millions every day on sexy novels, men's magazines, pornographic videos, and masturbatory sex aids, and even if each copy of *Playboy*, for example, was used as stimulus for only one act of masturbation, that would still add up to a couple of million acts of masturbation every month.

And even the sales figures of masturbatory aids don't take into account all of those men and women who masturbate using nothing more than their fingers and their own sexual fantasies to turn them on—men and women who would never think of buying a magazine or a sex-aid.

It isn't only single women who masturbate, either, by any means. Here's Hedwig, a 33-year-old home-maker from Portland, Oregon: "John and I are very happily married, and our sex life has always been very passionate and active. However, he lost his job as an insurance broker about 18 months ago, and his new job selling insurance means that he has to travel away from home, sometimes two to three days at a time, sometimes for a whole week, or even longer. When he first went away, I missed his companionship so much that I didn't think about sex. But when I became more accustomed to spending two and three nights on my own, I began to find that I thought about sex more and more. I began to feel irritable and depressed and I didn't know why. One night I had such a strong sexual dream. I dreamed that I was in France, for some reason, and that I was watching a cabaret in which a huge muscular black man was balancing a beautiful young white girl on his hand. She was dressed in nothing but a little ballet skirt. Her breasts were bare but covered with shiny silver spangles. The black man wore nothing but a sapphire satin pouch. His cock was only half-erect but it was enormous, and the pouch left nothing to the imagination. As he raised the girl up, she smiled at me, and gave me the strangest wink. It was then that I realized he was lifting her up with his fingers clasping her bottom and his thumb inserted into her pussy. The next thing I knew, I was lying in bed in my hotel, on my own. I knew that John had left me to go on business. I was nearly asleep when the comforter behind me was lifted up, and I felt somebody sliding into bed with me. I tried to turn around but I was held very tight—not roughly, but strongly. A voice said, 'Ssh,' and I knew that it was the black man from the cabaret. He was naked and his cock was fully erect. I could feel it bobbing against my bare back.

"He reached down between my legs so that he could open my pussy with his fingers. Then he pushed his cock into me, from behind. It slid in, and in, and in. It was so huge that I gasped out loud. I felt as if it wouldn't stop until it came out of my mouth. He took hold of the base of his cock and stirred it around, and my insides were churned around by this huge penis until I felt that I was going to have an orgasm even before we had started to fuck.

"He started to push in and out of me, and I remember screaming, in my dream, screaming with excitement, screaming with pleasure. I sometimes wonder if I was really screaming, out loud. I don't think that people do that, when they're asleep.

"He clasped my waist, and rolled onto his back, lifting me up so that I was on top of him, but facing upward. He reached down and stroked my bare thighs with fingers that felt like electricity. You see, it excites me just to remember it! He ran his fingertips up my sides, so that I shuddered, and then he touched my breasts and twisted my nipples between his fingers. He kept on giving me little, strong thrusts, his cock going in and out of me. He said, 'Reach down, and feel between your legs,' so I did. He said, 'You have a big pair of balls now, black balls.' And I reached down and felt these huge, tight wrinkled balls, right between my thighs, and my own wet pussy-lips, and my own clitoris, which was stiffer than I thought was possible. I started to stroke his balls and scratch them with the tips of my fingernails. I said, 'Your beautiful ball-bags, I'd like to lick them.' At the same time I started to stroke my clitoris . . . I've always liked to have my clitoris gently stroked downward with the side of my thumb, while I tickled myself with the tip of my index finger just above my pussy hole.

"He thrust and thrust, and I could hear him grunting underneath me, feel his hard chest muscles tightening, feel his hips rising. His balls seemed to swell enormously. I could feel them bulging, almost, as if they were filled up with boiling sperm. Then I had an orgasm—a spine-cracking orgasm that made me shake, and shake, it was almost *painful*. And of course I woke up, and I was alone in bed, sweating, the sheet *flooded* with juices in a way that I had never seen before. I thought I had wet the bed, but I hadn't. My thighs were tightly clamped together, and my hand was clamped between them. There had been no black man, but I *had* been masturbating.

"I got up and I showered, and of course I realized what had been happening to me. I used to have vivid sexual dreams when I was younger, but I hadn't had a dream like that since I first met John. The simple fact was that I was sexually frustrated. I badly needed a fuck.

"Two days later, I met an old friend of ours when I was out doing the marketing for the weekend. His name was Alan, and I was surprised to see him shopping on his own. I asked him if his wife Joyce was sick, and he said, no, he and Joyce were separated and they were going to divorce. He asked me to have a drink with him after we had finished up at the store, and of course I said yes. I didn't see any harm in it.

"But later, when we were in the cocktail lounge together, and chatting and laughing, it occurred to me Alan was a very attractive man, and that he obviously liked me, too, and that it would be very easy for us to go to bed together if we wanted to. I went to the rest-room and stared at myself in the mirror, and I was almost arguing with myself like those cartoon charac-ters sometimes do, with a little angel on one side of their head and a little devil on the other.

"Who would know, if Alan were to come home with me and we were to make love? And then I thought to myself: *I* would know, and I loved John, and just be-cause I was feeling frustrated, that was no reason to ruin our marriage.

"I decided no. And I decided something else—that it was time to tell John the way I felt. When he called me up from Spokane that evening, I took a deep breath and told him that I'd had a sexy dream. I said I loved him and I missed him, and those nights when he was away from me were pretty difficult to bear. I took an-other deep breath and told him that I'd masturbated.

"There was a moment's silence, but then I heard nothing in his voice but understanding. Understanding and *relief*, too, because the first thing he said was, 'You don't think that *I* haven't been masturbating, too?'

"Do you know something, that evening, we broke down an incredible barrier between us, a kind of un-spoken taboo that just because two people are married to each other, there won't be times when one or both of them feels like masturbating. We agreed that mas-turbation didn't amount to adultery, no way. In fact, under the circumstances that *we* were in, loving each other but being forcibly separated by economic neces-sity, masturbation was a declaration of faithfulness. It showed that we were both passionate and sexual peo-ple, and that we needed regular physical release, but that we didn't want to look for that physical release with anybody else.

"Things didn't look black from then on. John had to go out to dinner, but I called him back at bedtime. I showered and washed my hair and sprayed myself with his favorite perfume—Giorgio Red—not that *he* could smell it, of course, but I could. I lay back on the bed and I told him that I was wearing my black lacy bra and my black lacy panties and my black lacy garter belt and my black sheer stockings. I told him that I was pinching my nipples through my bra so that they stiffened up. Then I was taking off my bra, and massaging my bare breasts with my hand. Then I was reaching down my body, and sliding my hand inside my stocking tops.

"He said, 'I'm naked . . . I'm totally hard . . . I'm slowly rubbing my cock up and down . . .'

"I told him I was stroking my panties . . . they were damp already and the juice was glistening in the black lace. Then I was sliding my fingers inside, so that I could feel my swelled-up pussy lips, and my juicy insides. I pulled my panties to one side, so that my pussy was completely exposed. Now I was sliding two fingers inside me.

"I put the telephone down between my legs so that he could hear how juicy I was. In fact, I massaged it around and around against my pussy. Then I told him I was licking my own juice off the telephone, and blowing him kisses, too.

"I stroked my clitoris, and I tried to let him know how I was feeling, every single tingle. Then I couldn't speak to him any longer, I could only pant, but he was panting, too, because he was masturbating himself to a climax.

"We came almost together—the first time we'd come so close together for ages! It wasn't intercourse, but it was making love, and it released both of our tensions, and we did it together, and openly, instead of hiding it and feeling guilty about it.

"These days, whenever John goes away, masturbating on the telephone is part of our normal bedtime routine. He even bought me a huge vibrator in the shape of a man's penis, so that I can close my eyes and pretend that he's fucking me.

"The strange thing is, it's actually brought us closer together. I don't know why, but we seem to understand each other's needs a whole lot more, and I think quite honestly that John has become a much better lover."

The reasons for the improvement in John and Hedwig's lovemaking aren't difficult to find. First of all, their separation led to them putting the strength of their sexual desire for each other into words. It's surprising how few couples do this. Try to think, for instance, of the last time that *you* told a husband or lover "You turn me on," or said *anything* that let him know that you think he's sexy.

A failure to verbalize your sexual feelings is understandable, of course, especially in a long-term relationship in which you both feel familiar and comfortable, and which, to all intents and purposes, appears to be secure. Cara, 41, a legal assistant from New Orleans, told me: "I don't need to tell Burt that he excites me in bed. We've been married too long. I'd be embarrassed to say it, and Burt would wonder what in the blue blazes was wrong with me."

But in my experience, it's essential that you overcome your embarrassment about "talking sexy", and that you give your lover regular sexual compliments. "You know I love you" isn't good enough. Tell your lover how good looking he is. Tell him that he still has that animal magnetism that attracted you when you first met him. Tell him how big and virile his penis is. Tell him that when he makes love to you, you're in seventh heaven. Tell him you're so turned on that you think you're going to die.

Obviously you have to choose your moment. You wouldn't say, "Your cock is wonderful and enormous and I just love it when you slide it into me," just when you're paying for two bags of kitty litter at the supermarket checkout. But when you have a quiet, intimate moment together, tell him he's sexy . . . and if he hasn't already told you that *you* turn *him* on, tease him and coax him until he does, and make sure that he sees how pleased you are.

The second reason why John and Hedwig's relationship was so much improved was because when they masturbated over the telephone they were unable to see each other and had to explain *everything* they felt. This meant that they had to think about what they felt at each particular stage in their growing sexual excitement, and then describe it as accurately as possible. They also had to judge how excited their partner was at each particular stage . . . and what their partner was doing in order to accelerate or to slow down their approaching climax.

Was John rubbing his penis more slowly? Was he gripping the shaft tighter? Was he stimulating his testicles or his anus? And what about Hedwig? Was she directly massaging her clitoris? Was she caressing her breasts? Had she inserted one more finger into her vagina?

Over a period of weeks, they learned in considerable detail what to do when their partner wasn't quite as excited as they were, or was much *more* excited than they were. Where to kiss, where to lick, where to touch, *how* to touch. They acquired an unusually high degree of competence in those sexual skills that are required for a couple to make love with closely matching rhythms, and with closely matching levels of erotic excitement.

"We had never reached a climax together, not once," said Hedwig. "But suddenly we found that we could do it, almost whenever we wanted."

The third reason was that they had lost all of their inhibitions about discussing sex together. They had developed between them an easy, articulate language of love which, in my opinion, was one of the most valuable of all their newly acquired skills.

Many lovers have an urgent need to discuss their love life together but find it extremely difficult to put their thoughts into words. In school, we are taught the subtleties of describing "a snowy day" or "Thanksgiving dinner" or "my favorite feelings." But we are never taught how to discuss our sexual feelings. We are never equipped with the words to talk about "having my clitoris sucked" or "my most outrageous erotic fantasy." You can imagine the outcry from parents if a school *did* include such subjects in its curriculum!

Read any restaurant review, in any newspaper or magazine. It will be laden with adjectives . . . "Beef was well-hung tender and richly flavored, its sauce a subtle combination of sage and madeira; brill had a basil and mustard crust and another fine sauce of vermouth and red peppers." Yet any description of sexual behavior that was verbalized with such lip-licking relish would be considered embarrassing at best and pornographic at worst.

If you saw how many letters I receive from young women saying "I'd like to try oral sex, but what does sperm actually *taste* like?" or from men saying "I love going down on my wife, I love drinking the juice out of her when she climaxes, but the trouble is, she doesn't believe me, and I don't know how to convince her," then you would realize how prudish and limited our sexual vocabulary has become.

Sexual relationships are misfiring or breaking up every minute of the day, for no other reason than the fact that men and women are incapable of telling each other what they want and how they feel. I sat on the panel of *The Shirley Show* on Canadian television recently and encouraged the audience simply to say out loud what was worrying them about sex, and believe me, that audience could have gone on talking all night.

Talking about sex, using sexual words, finding a sexual vocabulary that enables men and women to express their appetites and their frustrations—that, to me, is one of the greatest priorities in sexual self-training.

The single woman who masturbates is doing nothing worse than enjoying the capacity for sexual pleasure with which she was born. Masturbation does no physical or emotional harm, nor does it diminish a single woman's ability to enjoy herself sexually when she *does* find a partner. The plain truth is that you can masturbate yourself day and night forever after and it will have no effect on you whatsoever, except to strengthen your fingers.

You can understand why masturbation was frowned upon in previous generations. Apart from a puritanical aversion to anything that smacked of pleasure for pleasure's sake, there were many small communities which depended on burgeoning populations simply to survive. Life expectancy was short, children died young. If a woman had a sexual urge, then it was best directed to getting herself pregnant.

But times have changed and society has changed. Millions of women find themselves now without lovers, husbands, or friends. Yet they still have sexual appetites, and to censure them for masturbation is not only physiologically, psychologically, and politically incorrect, it's totally unfair, too.

Every woman masturbates in her own individual way. Some of these methods of self-stimulation are really quite simple, but others are very elaborate indeed. I received a letter from a 45-year-old woman in Phoenix who had suspended two loops of twine from the guttering of her house, so that she could push her sunbed up against the wall, lift her ankles into the loops, and lie naked on her sunbed underneath her outside shower, its warm spray directed right onto her clitoris.

"I can close my eyes and I don't even have to touch myself."

Some women can reach orgasm simply by massaging their breasts and nipples, and not even touching themselves vaginally. However, the ability to do this regularly is very rare, and most women find that stimulating their breasts is an additional pleasure to clitoral masturbation rather than a substitute. Every act of masturbation is different, just as every act of sexual intercourse is different. Your level of excitement and your ultimate feeling of satisfaction (or lack of satisfaction) will depend on all kinds of factors, most of which will be beyond your control.

- How long since you last made love?
- What time of the month is it? (Are you just on the verge of starting a period?)
- Are you in love with a particular man at the moment?
- Does he turn you on?
- Do you currently have a new and exciting sexual fantasy?
- Are you anxious about anything in your personal life?
- Are you worried about your job/ your children/ your general security?
- Do you masturbate (a) frequently; (b) occasionally; (c) hardly ever?
- Do you feel guilty about this particular act of masturbation?
- Are you concerned that even if you don't feel guilty now you will almost certainly feel guilty afterward?

On the surface of it, it seems to be quite logical that you will be feeling more sexually frustrated if you haven't made love to a man in quite a long time, and that the longer you haven't done it, the more sexually frustrated you will be.

Although nobody has ever undertaken any serious research on the subject, it appears from my quarter-century of experience that women who are deprived of sex experience feelings of frustration that have very strong parallels with the feelings of women who give up smoking or alcohol or soft drugs.

First of all, they feel confident and brave about it. Then they start having doubts about it. Then they crave it, in a period of unbearable craving that may go on for months and months without letup. Then, suddenly, they don't think about it any more. Both physically and emotionally, their brains and their bodies have adapted to their new life patterns.

How long it takes for a woman to stop thinking constantly about sex will vary dramatically from woman to woman. I talked to a 49-year-old New York nun who confessed that she still had strong sexual feelings, and that for three years "I felt that I ought to beg for exorcism, because there was a devil in my soul."

But women who live without sex for a long period of time often grow to accept their celibacy, and in the place of sexual passion they often develop a new passion, such as art or music or charity work. Women without men are often the highest of the high flyers in industry and politics and law, presumably because they have diverted all of their sexual and emotional energies into their career. I have asked several of them if they would give up their success in exchange for sexual satisfaction. Their responses have ranged from "Absolutely not," to "No trade," to "Yes, I miss it, but I wouldn't give up my personal status and $117,000 a year for the sake of a few sweaty fucks"—to even, from one woman attorney, "The question never arises. Now that I'm financially independent, I can buy all of the sex that I want."

The interesting thing is, though, that out of 103 single professional women with whom I talked about sex and celibacy, 37 percent admitted that they masturbated "once a month, maybe more than once a month"; 28 percent admitted that they masturbated "more than once a month"; 26 percent admitted that they masturbated "once a week"; 17 percent said they masturbated "more than once a week"; 14 percent said "virtually every day". Only 4 percent maintained that they "never masturbated."

Remember that this wasn't a sample of *all* women, of all social classes and backgrounds. It was a small, elite group of women who have become successful in their careers and independent of husbands or lovers, both emotionally and financially. All the same, it was surprising how many of them consider that masturbation is a perfectly acceptable way for a single woman to release her sexual tensions.

Janice, 29, a redheaded accountant from Omaha, Nebraska, told me: "I started to masturbate when I was just a child. I can't remember a time when I haven't fingered myself just for the sheer pleasure of it. But I always used to feel so guilty about it. I didn't think that it was wrong until we had a talk on sex at school, when I was about 15. The woman who was giving the talk described masturbation as 'disgusting and degraded,' and said that girls who masturbated would never be able to achieve sexual satisfaction when they eventually got married because their sexual organs would be 'numbed' by so much fingering.

"Of course that really worried me. I managed to stop myself masturbating for a while, but it was close to exam time, and because I was so stressed and working so hard, I started up again.

"I first had sexual intercourse when I was 17, with a very handsome football player named Jake. He isn't a football player any longer—he's an accountant—but we're still friends. The way I felt when he touched me . . . well, that was just fantastic. I think I'm unusual in that I actually *enjoyed* losing my virginity. I knew then that the sex-talk woman had been talking hogwash, and that masturbation doesn't do you any harm at all. It didn't do *me* any harm, anyway. I sure wasn't 'numb'! The second time Jake made love to me, I had an orgasm, and then I had another orgasm, and another, and he was just beautiful.

"If you want my opinion, I think I enjoyed making love a whole lot more because masturbating had taught me so much about my feelings, and how to stimulate myself.

"I was married when I was 23. It didn't work out, but it was a compatibility problem, not a sexual problem. We divorced on my 27th birthday. Since then, I've had plenty of boyfriends, but I've been concentrating on building my career and enjoying myself. I collect antique jewelry and American primitive paintings and I love music. You don't think Omaha has music? You should come to the Orpheum Theater!

"I masturbate because I like it and because it's harmless and because it *does* relieve those feelings of sexual frustration. What really turns me on is to masturbate outside, in the open air. Some nights I take off all of my clothes and go into the yard at the back of the house. It's very private—the neighbors can't see very much of it. I lie on the garden swing, completely naked, and look up at the stars and listen to the sound of next door's TV, or people talking, or music, or traffic, and I play with my nipples. I've always had real sensitive nipples. When I was young I could actually reach an orgasm just by pinching my nipples, but I haven't been able to do that in quite a while.

"Sometimes I clip clothespins on my nipples, or earrings. It's just a little extra turn-on, having my nipples pinched. I don't think I'm masochistic. I wouldn't like to have my nipples pierced, or anything like that. But I did once meet a girl who had a diamond stud in her pussy lips, and I thought that was such a turn-on I seriously thought about having it done myself.

"I masturbate with both hands. I like to flick my clitoris upward with the middle finger of my right hand—very quickly, scarcely touching it. With my other hand, I reach underneath my bottom, and I insert my index finger and my middle finger into my pussy, and my thumb into my ass. All the time that I'm flicking my clitoris with my right hand, I'm rhythmically squeezing the fingers of my left hand together. I close my eyes and feel the night breeze blowing over me, and I'm in heaven.

"I would guess that it doesn't take me more than six or seven minutes to reach orgasm. Do I fantasize? Sometimes, but my fantasies are more abstract than anything else. I have a favorite fantasy in which I'm a slave girl and I'm never allowed to wear clothes, and any man who wants to touch me or fuck me can do it whenever he feels like it. I might be bending down to pick up a plate, and a man can push his finger into my ass, and I simply have to remain bending, and completely cooperative, until he's finished.

"I'm not a submissive person. Not at all. In fact, my friends seem to think that I'm pretty fiery. But I guess we all have fantasies in which we're sexually dominated."

Janice, of course, is quite right. Many people have erotic fantasies in which they're helpless or submissive. Such fantasies relieve us of any responsibility for our sexual conduct, and (particularly for men) they neatly sidestep the fear of sexual failure. Read any pornographic magazine for men and you will see that more often than not the sexual acts that they describe do *not* involve violence or sexual coercion by men against women. In male pornography, in fact, it's very rarely the man who makes any kind of running at all. It's the women who make all the advances. The men don't have to risk being rebuffed. They don't have to take the blame for clumsy or incompetent technique, or for failing to bring their partner to a climax, or for failing to keep their erection.

Similarly, in women's erotic fiction, it's the men who pick up the women and carry them helplessly into the bedroom, and then have their wicked way with them. The woman has to do nothing except weakly protest while her panties are torn off and his "engine of love" is forced between her legs.

Remember that just because you have fantasies about extreme sexual behavior when you're masturbating, that doesn't mean for a moment that you would act out such behavior in real life or that you're in any way "perverted."

Fantasy is fantasy, and for most well-adjusted people that's *all* it is. It's a way of stimulating ourselves mentally as well as physically; it does us no more harm than watching an exciting movie or reading a gripping novel.

SIX

Where the Toys Are

Apart from the highly stimulating combination of fingers and fantasy, there is a mind-boggling selection of sex toys on the market that can improve and intensify a single woman's masturbation. All of them are available mail order (which means that you won't have to face the embarrassment of buying them over the counter). You will usually find advertisements for sex-toy catalogs in the back pages of *Playboy* or other men's magazines.

The best-selling sex toy ever is Joni's Butterfly (or variations of it). This is a butterfly-shaped vibrator of pink vinyl that a woman straps over her vulva with four elastic bands. It has a "clitoral stimulator," an "anal tantalizer," and four rows of "stimulating nodules." All a woman has to do is switch it on and the butterfly will "fly and flutter its tantalizing vibrations throughout her vaginal area." The intensity of the vibrations can be controlled with a hand-held switch. The advertisement for Joni's Butterfly says: "WARNING: Once strapped into position and activated there is no escape from the pleasurable sensations."

Roxanne, a 33-year-old secretary from Pittsburgh, reported: "I didn't like the look of Joni's Butterfly very much. It reminded me of one of those old-fashioned sanitary belts. Unlike your ordinary penis-shaped vibrator, which you can just keep under your pillow, or in your nightstand drawer, and slip out when you feel like it, I very much had the feeling that I was preparing myself for masturbation, and that was off-putting. I'm not ashamed of masturbating. What else can you do when you don't have a lover? But I definitely had an uncomfortable feeling when I put on Joni's Butterfly . . . not exactly inadequacy, not exactly embarrassment, but it was a little bit like being on your own at Christmas, and using a special clamp to hold one end of a cracker so that you can pull it with yourself.

"However, when I did strap it on and started it going, I have to say that the feeling was sensational. It certainly gets nine out of ten for turning you on! It sets up a gentle, persistent vibration that gave me an absolutely unique tingle between my legs . . . I had never felt anything like it, ever. It took me a long time to reach an orgasm, but I think that was mainly because I wasn't used to it and I did have a certain amount of consumer resistance to something that looked so much like a surgical appliance.

"The first orgasm came quite unexpectedly . . . it just rose up inside me and the next thing I knew I was gripping the sheets and quaking about 6 on the Richter scale. Then I had another, and another, and another. I had never in my life had four orgasms one after the other, and by the time I was finished I felt exhausted. I guess I could have gone on, and had more, because the great thing about Joni's Butterfly is that it doesn't get tired, and it doesn't roll over and go to sleep just when you need it the most. All you need is batteries.

"I'm a convert now. I like it because I can wear it under my pajamas and switch it on whenever I'm feeling a little bit horny."

Even what Roxanne described as "your ordinary penis-shaped vibrator" has gone through a dramatic transformation. Modern latex technology and the introduction of new plastic materials has meant that the old hard rocket-shaped vibrator of days gone by has been replaced by enormously sophisticated and detailed vibrators that are barely distinguishable from real penises—except that they vibrate, and they don't have a man on the end.

You can still buy the straightforward rocket shape, but these days it's equipped with a whole variety of extra attachments. The "Horny Foreplay Kit," for example, contains a basic vibrator and all of these gadgets which can be fitted over the end of it: (a) a soft cup shape for stimulating nipples, (b) a soft bud shape for clitoral vibration, (c) a curved dildo for so-called "G-Spot" stimulation, (d) a thin finger for anal vibration, (e) a soft brush for "all-over" tingling.

In the "lifelike" department, there is a huge selection of vibrating penises to choose from. The Swinger is a vibrator "which has been designed for discerning ladies who need the real feel of a good stiff penis deep inside them. This fleshy latex dildo is a fully-erect 22 centimeters long, with a slightly curved shaft and a superbly realistic helmet."

Then there's Buck Bronson's 10-inch Penis, produced by taking a plaster-cast of porno star Buck Bronson's enormous penis, which hangs down almost to his knees. "It's manufactured from the most realistic fleshy material which even sweats like a real penis on a boner." It has "real-feel" testicles that actually move, and—when squeezed—it actually ejaculates.

One of the best-selling vibrators in the world is the "Bully Boy," a thick, curved penis with a variable-speed vibrating motor. Apart from its thickness, the "Bully Boy's" most distinctive feature is its base, which has "titillating projecting nodules." It's available in pink or black, depending on the color that you want your fantasy lover to be!

The "Deep Stroker" is a penis that actually concertinas up and down when you switch it on. The "Tri-Star Pleaser" has three vibrating clitoral stimulators protruding from its base, so that the deeper you push it in, the more your clitoris is massaged.

Another best seller is "Mr. Softy," a dildo made of pliable plastic material that "looks, feels and acts just like a solid hot penis that's hungry for sex." Other dildoes actually light up at the end, or have a heat element which warms them up "to the temperature of an erect penis," whatever that is.

Among some oversized dildoes are the "Taras Bulba," which you can pump up with air once it's inside your vagina, to make it as big as you like—"it swells to bursting in order to please you." Then there's "Big Jock," over 25 centimeters long—"insert with care increasing to full vibro-power slowly when you're sure you can stand it." "Thor the Mighty" is "26 centimeters of throbbing joy—incedibly realistic, right down to the veins which have been enhanced to increase the arousing effect."

In recent years, anal stimulation has "come out of the closet," and anal dildoes and "butt plugs" are openly advertised. The smallest of these is a three-tier vibrator with a specially wide base. The most amusing is a dildo shaped like a small fist, which punches furiously from side to side when you switch it on. The largest is the "Anal Goliath," a huge 40-centimeter plastic penis with a handle that makes it look more like a sword, designed for "gigantic anal stimulation."

Other anal stimulators include the "Anal Prober," a thin, flexible vibrator with a bulb-shaped nodule on the end, for exploring deep inside your bottom; the "Anal Placator," a curved, knobbly anal dildo; or the "Anal Pounder," a miltispeed anal vibrator with a screw thread.

Some single women feel that dildoes and vibrators are demeaning—particularly those women who have chosen to live without men, rather than those women who have been divorced or separated, or who haven't yet met "Mr. Perfect."

Sara, 25, a welfare worker from Sacramento, wrote: "I am a normal, loving woman who has no problem at all with sexual hang-ups. However, I would never consider masturbating with an inanimate object such as a vibrator. If I cannot have a real penis then I certainly do not want a plastic one! It really is the height of male arrogance to manufacture artificial penises for women who for very good reasons do not have access to real ones. Why don't they make artificial vaginas for single men?"

As a matter of fact, of course, they *do* have artifical vaginas, of every conceivable shape and size and variety, from the full-blown artificial woman made of solid latex to the inflatable woman (footpump extra) to "Pussy Galore." ("Take a little piece of me home tonight! I can offer you two versions of my sweet vagina which, I am assured, will grab you just like my real one on which they were modelled. Both with pump action to simulate orgasm.")

But although I can understand Sara's point of view, I don't really think that it's "male arrogance" that prompts the manufacture and sale of dildoes and other sex toys for women. They *do* sell, and in quite staggering quantities. More dildoes are bought by men than most sex toy retailers like to suggest, but the fact remains that thousands and thousands are bought by single women, as a straightforward aid to masturbation.

And why not? They're clean, harmless, pleasurable, and undemanding . . . and when you've finished with them you can shut them in the wardrobe and forget about them. More than you can do with a man.

Here's Angela, a 26-year-old divorcée from Austin, Texas: "We had a party around at one of my friend's houses about a year ago, when they were selling sexy lingerie. I bought a satin teddy, which I really liked, and which I still wear in the evenings sometimes, when I'm alone at home. I also bought a set of three different G-strings, which are great for wearing under jeans or slacks because they don't give you any visible panty line. But the girl also gave us a couple of mail-order catalogs to take away, and when I got them home that evening and read them, I found that one of them was filled with all kinds of sex toys, such as vibrators and dildoes and some things that I'd never even heard of.

"I saw a dildo in the catalog called 'Mr. Softy.' The advertisement said that it felt just like a real man's penis. I looked at it again and again, and when I was in bed that night I thought about it some more, and turned myself on so much that I masturbated. Up until then, I didn't use objects when I masturbated. I knew some girls at high school who masturbated with shampoo bottles or hairbrush handles. There was one girl named Susan who always used to masturbate with the handle of a baseball bat, with a condom on it and everything!

"But the way I always masturbated, I used to lie back naked on the bed with my legs very wide open. Then I stretched apart my pussy lips with my left hand and fingered my clitoris with my right hand. As I got more and more excited, I bunched all of the fingertips of my left hand together, and dipped them quickly in and out of my open pussy. I always did it like that, but I guess every woman has a different way of doing it. I had never thought of using a penis substitute before.

"I resisted buying 'Mr. Softy' for nearly a month. Then one night I had a dream that I had bought one and that I was pushing it slowly into my pussy. The feeling was so ecstatic that I was moaning and crying. In fact, I was moaning and crying so much that I woke myself up. I lay awake for over an hour, and while I was lying there, I thought to myself: This is ridiculous. You're a grown woman, you can do what you like. If you want an artificial penis, then for God's sake buy yourself an artificial penis. Who's going to know?

"So the next day I called the mail-order people and ordered 'Mr. Softy.' The girl who took my order was completely unfazed. She made me feel as if ordering a plastic penis was the most natural and normal thing in the world. And, of course, if you're a single woman who doesn't have a lover, but you still enjoy the feeling of a fat cock inside you—and what woman *doesn't,* even if it's only occasionally—then ordering a plastic penis *is* the most natural and normal thing in the world.

"The girl even asked me if I wanted the seven-inch or the eight-inch version, and when I asked her what *she* thought, she said, 'The eight-inch is ten dollars more, ma'am, but it's worth every cent.'

" 'Mr. Softy' arrived three or four days later in a padded envelope. I opened him up and there he was, stiff but bendy, shiny and pink, complete with a big fat penis-shaped head on him, and veins all the way down his shaft. I couldn't use him then and there, because I was late for work, but I thought about him all day. When I went to the washroom halfway through the morning, I found that my pussy was flooded with juice and that my panties were soaking. I was almost tempted to masturbate right there, in the washroom. But I decided to wait until I got home, and use 'Mr. Softy.'

"When I arrived home, I went through to the bedroom and undressed immediately. 'Mr. Softy' was waiting for me where I had left him, under my pillow. I lay back on the bed and opened up my legs and started to touch myself in the usual way, opening up my pussy lips and fingering my clitoris. Then I couldn't hold myself back any longer. I reached under the pillow and took out 'Mr. Softy'. He was surprisingly warm and lifelike . . . there was nothing cold and plasticky about him at all. I nudged his head between my legs, and then I made him bounce gently against my open pussy. All the time I kept on fingering and rubbing my clitoris, and my pussy was so juicy that it was making a sticky kind of squelching noise every time I rubbed it.

"I lifted up my head so that I could see what I was doing really clearly. I opened up my pussy lips wide, and then I slowly plunged 'Mr. Softy's' head into my open hole. All the time my fingertips were slithering around and around my clitoris, which was sticking out like a little pink bird's beak. I pushed 'Mr. Softy' in further, and then pulled him out an inch or two, then pushed him back in again. I was rubbing my clitoris quicker and harder, and a feeling was growing inside me like a volcano that's about to erupt.

"I turned around on the bed so that I could see myself in the dressing-table mirror. My pussy lips were swollen and flushed, and my pussy hair was all stuck together, because it was so wet. 'Mr. Softy' went right inside me, all eight inches of him, and when I pulled him out, my hole was still in the shape that it had been when he was inside of me, a perfect circle; and *he* was all slippery with juice.

"I pushed him in and out of me faster and faster and rubbed my clitoris faster. It was a totally fantastic feeling. It wasn't like being fucked by a man, but it gave me the same kind of physical excitement, and it gave me something else, too—a feeling of freedom, that I was a grown woman who could do anything she liked, no matter how 'dirty' it was, and that I was completely in control of my own sexual pleasure.

"As I got close to having a climax, I pushed 'Mr. Softy' in and out much more slowly, and squeezed him tight with my pussy muscles so that I could feel every inch of him, his head, and his veins, and his big rubbery shaft.

"I had one of those climaxes where everything goes dark, and then you're jumping and kicking around the bed, and thrashing your arms, and there's nothing you can do to stop yourself. I stirred 'Mr. Softy' around and around inside my pussy until I had gotten the last ounce of pleasure out of that climax, and then I lay back with my eyes closed, feeling deliciously satisfied, and slowly, slowly sliding him in and out of me.

"What I really like about 'Mr. Softy' is that I can keep him inside of me all night if I want to. All I have to do is slide him up me and then put on a tight pair of pants which prevents me from squeezing him out. It's just like having a man's stiff cock inside me from morning till night . . . which, of course, a real man could never do! I've done it twice now, and the second time I masturbated eight times, all through the night.

"I may not have a lover, but I do get plenty of sex."

Angela was typical of many single women who try dildoes or other sex toys for masturbation. At first, almost all of them felt that the use of a dildo was somehow demeaning or shameful, an admission that they had been unable to attract a real man with a real penis.

But there is nothing shameful about using a dildo. It is simply an aid to giving you sexual pleasure, and for relieving sexual tensions. Candice, 28, an airline flight attendant from Charleston, South Carolina, said: "I have a vibrator, for sure, and I masturbate, yes. It's no substitute for sex with a man, but it does take off the sexual pressure when I'm in between boyfriends. I sometimes think that I would have made one or two really serious mistakes in dating men if I hadn't been so cool, calm, and collected. And that's what masturbation allows me to be. I'm not forever prowling around, desperate for a cock, which some of my friends are."

Renata, a 40-year-old divorcée from Cleveland, said: "My marriage broke up because of my lack of sexual expertise. I was taught very little about sex when I was a girl. My mother was mortally embarrassed by any mention of sex, although when I was 14 she left a booklet on childbirth on my pillow, with a note saying, 'Hope this helps!'

"I had a very sympathetic teacher at school who gave me honest and straightforward answers to all of my questions about sex. But that wasn't enough. When you're learning about sex, you need more than answers, because most of the time you don't even know the questions. How are you expected to ask about multiple orgasms when you don't even know that you can have single orgasms? How are you expected to ask how a woman can really enjoy anal sex when you didn't even know that anal sex existed?

"The breakup of my marriage was my husband's fault as much as mine. I had been living in a blissful state of ignorance for seven years, thinking that our sex life was wonderful because Maurice got on top of me two or three times a week. To tell you the truth, I didn't enjoy sexual intercourse all that much, but I was happy because Maurice seemed to be happy, and I loved holding him close, and having him kiss me.

"He used to caress my anus sometimes when we were making love, and I didn't mind that. Occasionally he tried to push his finger into it, but I always used to react by squeezing my muscles very tight and pressing the cheeks of my bottom together so that he couldn't do it.

"He used to try to kiss me between the legs, but I didn't like the idea of that either, and whenever he went down on me I used to turn to one side so that he couldn't do it. I knew men got very passionate when they were making love, and my mother had warned me that men would always 'try things.' But she said that 'you don't have to do what you don't want to do . . . you don't have to do anything that isn't proper.'

"Well, of course, being so green I thought that it wasn't proper for a man to kiss my vagina and it wasn't proper for a man to stick his finger up my bottom. I didn't even realize until divorce proceedings had started that my husband had also been trying to coax me into giving him oral sex. I always used to wonder why he kept sitting up in bed when we were watching television together, with his cock so close to my face. I used to cover it over with the comforter and tell him not to show off!

"You wouldn't think it, but I'm a very sexual person. Well, I am now—now that I've discovered my sexuality.

"My husband left me for a girl who worked in his office. She was pretty, but she wasn't any prettier than me. She had a good figure, but I've got much bigger breasts, and Maurice always said that he loved big breasts. When I asked him cold why he wanted her more than he wanted me, he said, 'You were frigid.' Which totally stunned me. Can you imagine your husband saying that to your face after seven years of what *you* thought was a happy, active sex life?

"He said, 'She does everything that you never did.' And I said, 'What did I never do? Tell me!' But he wouldn't. He wouldn't even give me the chance to find out what it was that I had never done, and to try doing it.

"I was very depressed for a while. Then I picked up one of your books, *How to Drive Your Man Wild in Bed*. It was a complete eye-opener. I felt so embarrassed that I had known so little about sex and lovemaking. I suddenly realized what Maurice had wanted; and why he must have felt so frustrated.

"I decided to find out what I was really capable of, sexually, the way you suggest in your book. I groomed myself, I went to the hair salon, I had a manicure. I had my legs waxed and I had my whole bikini area waxed, too. I just love my new bare-look vagina! I had a massage to get all the kinks out of my muscles. I looked in the mirror every morning, completely naked, and I said to myself, 'You're beautiful.' And I believe it. And I was determined that somebody else was going to believe it, too.

"I went through all of that self-discovery routine that you recommend—exploring my sexual feelings by touching myself, exploring myself in front of the mirror. Opening up my vagina so that I could see right inside, to see what it looked like, to see what shape it was. I never used to touch myself sexually when I was younger . . . I don't know why. Maybe my mother discouraged it. But to spend an hour or two in front of a mirror, with my legs open wide, touching and stroking myself, seeing what happens when I get sexually excited, seeing where my clitoris is, seeing the hole that I piss out of (I was 31 and I'd never actually seen it before!)—all of that was wonderful and enlightening and made me feel attractive again, and sexual again, and womanly again, which is exactly how you *don't* feel after your husband has just left you for another girl.

"I masturbated with my fingers for a while, but I didn't find it very satisfactory, and I could never reach a climax. Maybe that was because I had never masturbated when I was a teenager, and the only times that I had ever reached a climax was when Maurice was making love to me. I missed the feeling of having a penis inside my vagina, that was all.

"I did like you suggested and bought a vibrator. I don't know what it's called, but it's very big, bigger than a real penis. What really sold me on it, though, was the fact that it had a foreskin, and, of course, Maurice is Jewish and circumcized and I was *fascinated* by the idea of a penis with a foreskin. Guess what it was called? 'The Giant Gentile'!

"I went to bed that night and pushed the vibrator up inside my vagina. I slid it in and out a few times, because I loved the way the foreskin rolled and unrolled. Then I switched it on—and I had *never* felt anything like it before. It turned me on so much that

I had to take it out. Then I had an idea, based on something that you mentioned in your book. I smothered my 'Giant Gentile' in KY, and I turned over on my side, and very gently I pushed the head of it up against my anus.

"I didn't really think I was going to be able to get it in. It felt so enormous and my anus felt so tight! But you said that if I pushed against the vibrator, my muscles would open, and so they did. I pushed hard, and my anus opened up, and slid this huge slippery dildo right up into my bottom, right up to the very end, where it was too wide for me to get it any further inside.

"I switched on the vibrator and I felt as if my *soul* was vibrating. I think I must have had an orgasm in less than a minute, and then another one, although that was smaller. That was the very first time I had ever put anything up inside my bottom, and I loved it! I lay back, with the vibrator still up inside me, and gently ran my fingertips around and around my anus. My anus was red and a little bit sore, but I loved the ticking sensation. I couldn't believe that my bottom had stretched open so wide . . . but here was the handle of this huge dildo sticking out of it. I suddenly realized that I *could* have let Maurice push his finger up inside it—he could even have pushed his cock up inside it. If only I'd known . . .

"I enjoyed my vibrator so much that I bought another, and now I usually masturbate with two. I don't have to do much. I slide one up inside my bottom, and the other inside my vagina, and switch them on to full vibrate. Then I press one fingertip against my clitoris, and that's enough to give me an orgasm within two to three minutes, maximum.

"I've learned a lot about myself, sexually. I've learned that I can reach my first orgasm quite quickly if I'm well stimulated, but then I'm always ready for another, deeper orgasm. I've learned that I like to have a penis angled slightly upward in my vagina, so that it presses against the front of my vagina. I've learned that I *do* enjoy anal stimulation while I'm making love . . . in fact, I'd like to have a vibrator up inside my bottom while a man's actually having sex with me. I bet that would blow his mind!

"There are some things you *can't* do with a vibrator. You can't practice oral sex. But now that I'm beginning to liberate myself sexually, I dream about doing that, too—*and* having it done to me. I long to feel a man's tongue inside my vagina, and I long to feel a man's hard penis inside my mouth."

A month after telling me about her masturbation techniques, Renata met a man two years her junior at a square dance, and started a relationship with him that, after two and a half weeks of dating, developed into sexual intimacy.

Her report: "This relationship is absolutely wonderful, not at all like my relationship with Maurice. I am really letting myself go, and together David and I are doing all the things that you mentioned in your book— and more!! David says that I am without a doubt the sexiest woman that he has ever met. I don't know whether marriage is on the horizon, but I am sure we are going to have a very happy time together, no matter what the outcome!"

So, apart from being very pleasurable, masturbation can also be very educational. Women who have never stimulated themselves sexually can often find difficulty in communicating to their lovers the ways in which they can be most quickly and intensely aroused. Often, once they *have* tried masturbation, they discover a new way of turning themselves on that never occurred to them before.

Jenny, a 23-year-old fashion model from Oakland, California, found out when she started masturbating that she was very rapidly aroused if she rhythmically pressed and tugged down with her fingers on the outer lips of her vulva, as well as quickly and lightly flicking her clitoris.

What she was doing, in fact, was pulling down on the muscles that run down on either side of the vulva. These muscles join together just above the vaginal opening to form the "arch" in which the clitoris is located. So each downward tug had a pulling effect on the deeply buried shaft of the clitoris, which added to the flicking sensation on the tip.

This masturbation technique can very effectively be used during intercourse, especially if the man has entered from the side or from behind. He can reach around during lovemaking and apply that same rhythmic tugging to your outer lips. Many women have found that this helps them to reach orgasm more quickly, and also gives a "deeper" quality to their orgasm when it actually occurs.

While you're masturbating, take some time to locate what is sometimes known as your "G-spot." In actual fact, there is no magical spot that, when stimulated, gives a woman an instant orgasm—which is why I always try to avoid using the term "G-spot." Your "G-spot" is simply the place where your vaginal wall is closest to the base of your clitoris.

Your clitoris is not just a little tip protruding from the top of your vulva. This is simply the glans of a highly sensitive organ that is buried beneath your skin just above it. The clitoris varies in size from woman to woman, just as the penis varies in size from man to man, but it averages about an inch long. You should be able to feel the shaft of it quite easily.

If you insert two fingers into your vagina and feel the front of your vaginal wall, you should be able to locate your clitoris from inside. This may not be terribly easy, depending on the length of your fingers and the location of your clitoris, and you may find it more effective if you use a dildo instead. You can buy specially curved dildoes that you can use to increase the pressure on the front of your vaginal wall during masturbation.

As you press rhythmically on your "G-spot," you may be able to feel your clitoris swelling and hardening—but don't worry if you can't. Depending on their anatomy, some women enjoy quite strong pressure on their "G-spot," while others can only tolerate a gentle stimulus.

The best way of massaging your "G-spot" is to have your lover do it for you. Lie back on the bed and open your legs wide, so that your lover can insert his two middle fingers deep into your vagina. If he bends his fingers so that his fingertips press against the front of your vaginal wall, he should be able to find your most sensitive place quite easily.

Many women report that having their "G-spot" stimulated has given them very strong and satisfying orgasms. There's certainly no harm in trying to locate it. Even if you *can't*, you'll have a great deal of erotic enjoyment in the process.

One result of massaging your "G-spot" during masturbation or intercourse is that your flow of vaginal juices may be greatly increased. In fact, some women produce such a flow of juice during a "G-spot" orgasm that they think they have wet the bed. When this happens, it's usually called a "wet orgasm"; you will easily be able to tell that you *haven't* wet the bed by the smell and consistency of the fluid that flows out of you.

Since the beginning of recorded time, there have been some quite staggering myths about how much fluid a woman produces during orgasm. Here, for example, is an excerpt from a Victorian erotic novel entitled *Sport Among the She-Noodles*:

'Ah, if mam only knew,' she sighed, as I was now sucking her titties, and running my disengaged hand up her thighs; they were nipped tightly together, but gradually relaxed under the pressure of my hand, till I actually got possession of her cunny, which I could feel was slightly covered with soft downy hair, and soon began to frig her gently with my forefinger. How the dear girl wriggled under this double excitement, and I could feel one of her hands groping outside my trousers over my bursting prick to return the pleasure that I was giving her. One by one she unfastened the buttons, then her soft delicate hand soon had possession of my stiff affair, naked and palpitating with unsatisfied desire.

'Ah,' she whispered, 'I am satisfied at last! We had a servant at home, a few months ago, who slept in our room, and used to tickle and play with us. She told us that men had a long thing as hard as iron, which they pleased the ladies by shoving up their bellies, and that was how babies were made. Do you believe it? She was always shoving her fingers into us as you are doing now, and, and—' here she hesitated and seemed to shudder with delight, just as I spent all over her hand, and I could also feel her spendings come in a warm gush all over my fingers.

If she were to read *that,* any woman would assume that her own vaginal juices were woefully inadequate, and any man would be likely to feel that he wasn't arousing his lover very well.

But the myth of female ejaculation continues, even today. Here's an extract from a brand-new erotic memoir, published in *Playbirds* magazine: "I ran the tips of my fingers over Kate's pussy lips as she lay there. Janet had been licking at Kate's pussy so those lips were nice and wet. I rubbed for a few seconds and then pushed two fingers into Kate's tight hole. She was soaking wet in there.

"I wanked them both hard and fast, and then, after I had taken my fingers out, Janet licked Kate's juices from one of my hands and then Kate licked Janet's juice from my other hand. Janet then got off the bed and left the room. I went down on Kate and sucked and licked at her wet pussy hole. I poked my tongue deep into the limits of her hole and no matter how much of her juice I managed to slurp out she always managed to produce more.

"Janet came back into the room, in her hand was a beer glass. Kate hunkered down with her thighs spread and almost at once large drops of her pussy juice began to dribble down from her pussy hole. Janet gave a sigh of desire and she held the beer glass under Kate so that the dribbles of pussy juice coming down from Kate's cunny tunnel went into it. The hot sweet scent of both their juices filled the room. More and more juice dribbled down into the glass, some of it was sort of frothing up in there. Then they changed places!

"Janet hunkered down, thighs spread, and Kate held the glass there, while Janet rubbed at her own clit and then it was Janet's juices that were bubbling and gurgling down into the glass and joining Kate's juices that were already there.

"The juices mixed and mingled, and soon that glass was half full, and Kate then took, it out from under Janet, and she smiled at me, and she lifted it to her mouth and took a long sip of it. Janet then took the glass, that glass filled with a thick scented mixture of Janet's juices and Kate's juices, and she took a long swallow from it.

"They were having orgasms as they passed it to each other, in fact after each sip they climaxed. They offered me the glass, and I took a sip. I was amazed. It was a sight I would remember for all time."

Apart from being appallingly badly written, this (genuine) extract is also appallingly inaccurate. As if there weren't already enough myths and misconceptions about sex, a magazine that purports to be "sexually liberated" has perpetuated the hoary old idea that women ejaculate fluid in copious quantities whenever they reach an orgasm. I suspect that the writer was genuinely ignorant about female physiology—but if he wasn't, then he deserves to be hung up by his thumbs.

Sex is wonderfully exciting without the need for gross exaggeration. I'm not anti-pornography. As a former editor of *Penthouse* and *Penthouse Forum* and the Swedish sex magazine *Private,* I have been able to see for myself that well-produced and informative erotica is positively beneficial: It links sound sexual information with intense sexual pleasure. A comprehensive knowledge of sex and sexual technique is a prerequisite for a happy, stimulating, and harmonious relationship, and so I *don't* appreciate it when writers create or perpetuate myths.

Unlike our performance in golf or tennis or swimming or any other leisure activity, we have no way of comparing our sexual performance with that of other people. That is why even the hardest of pornographers has something of a duty to stick to the possible, even if he is writing about the improbable. I have lost count of the number of anxious letters I have received from women worried about the flow of their vaginal juices. One woman wrote: "I can't manage to 'come' nearly as much as my husband, and this makes me feel as if I'm far less sexual than he is."

Through masturbation and self-exploration, you will begin to discover more and more about the way in which your body reacts to sexual stimulus. If you manage to locate your so-called "G-spot" and masturbate yourself to orgasm, you may very well find that you produce much more vaginal juice than usual, but it will still be far short of the quantity required to fill a beer glass!

Many men and women, however, do find that copious wetness is highly erotic (otherwise nobody would write pornographic stories about floods of vaginal juice or gallons of sperm.) Those people who are thrilled by wetness often add to their sexual pleasure by urinating while they masturbate or make love. "Wet sex" is a far more common practise than you would think from reading most of the standard manuals on sex. Thousands of ordinary and well-balanced lovers indulge in it, from playing with their partner's genitals while they urinate, to urinating all over each other's bodies and faces, and even drinking each other's urine.

I have received more letters about my candid and open discussion of wet sex than any other sexual topic, apart from impotence. Yet many sex manuals still classify it under "deviant behavior"—if they discuss it at all.

The simple fact is that thousands of lovers enjoy "wet sex" together, and many single men and women urinate as part of sexual self-stimulation. It's not a dirty practice. Fresh urine is completely sterile, and there are some health addicts who actually believe that it is beneficial to drink your own urine.

It is not uncommon for women to expel a little urine during orgasm, especially if they have a full bladder, and many men actually enjoy it when it happens. Dorothy, a 32-year-old sales assistant from Dallas, said: "My husband Joe thinks it's a real turn-on if I pee when I come. It's not much more than a single, quick spurt, but he loves it. He likes to go down on me, and give me an orgasm by licking my clitoris and sticking his tongue up inside my pussy. But what he likes most of all is when I actually come, and I shoot out a little spurt of pee, right onto his tongue. He says that I taste like nectar. He had a glass of whiskey once, and he wanted me to pee into it, so that he could find out what Rebel Yell and pee tasted like, but I was shy and I wouldn't. But one day I might. The idea of it doesn't disgust me at all. I used to be very embarrassed about peeing when I came, but Joe made me think of it as normal. In fact, he made me think that it was downright sexy, and that did my confidence no end of good."

Andrea, a 24-year-old shoe-store assistant, has been living alone for over a year since the break-up of her three-year relationship with Eddie.

"I masturbated a whole lot when I was a teenager. There was a group of five of us, sometimes six. We used to go around to each other's houses after school and read out all the sexy bits from books like *Scruples* and *Fear of Flying,* and try to imagine what it was going to be like to be fucked. While we were doing it, we used to take off their panties and openly masturbate. Sometimes we did it with candles or cucumbers, but mostly just our fingers, and sometimes we used to masturbate each other. I used to like that, masturbating another girl, feeling up her wet slippery cunt with my fingers, and I still fantasize about it sometimes, not that I'm a lesbian or anything like that. It was the fact that it was dirty and forbidden that made it exciting, that was all.

"We got into pissing, too. We used to go out for long walks together, and if we felt like taking a piss, we used to do it standing up, so that the others could watch, and sometimes we used to piss without taking our panties off. I used to like it when I pissed in my panties, and another girl slipped her hand inside and played with my cunt while I pissed.

"I enjoy pissing now, when I masturbate. I usually do it in the tub, with the plug in. I lie back and open my legs and stroke my cunt lips with my right hand, and press down on my pubic hair with my left hand. I don't like touching my clitoris directly—I find it too irritating. It's enough for me to trail my fingertips up and down my cunt lips, and keep pressing down on my pubic hair.

"When I start feeling seriously turned on, I press down on my bladder as well as my pubic hair, and after a while I piss. I pull my cunt lips apart so that I can watch it spraying out, and I like to tickle my piss hole while I'm doing it. Usually it sprays everywhere—all over my thighs and between my legs and runs down my stomach. I massage my whole body with warm piss—my breasts and my thighs—and I wash my face with it, too.

"I like to fantasize that I have a lover standing over me, and that he's holding his cock and pissing all over me. I have such a strong fantasy about a handsome man pissing in my hair, and all over my face. I'd love to take a man's cock in my mouth, so that he could piss down my throat.

"It doesn't take me long to reach a climax after I've pissed. Afterwards I always feel ashamed of myself, and empty the tub quickly, and give myself a thorough wash. I was so guilty about doing it once that I talked to my best friend Moira about it, and asked her if I needed to see a shrink. But she said that if I needed to see a shrink, then she did, too. She didn't have quite so many fantasies about pissing as I did, but she said that she'd watched her husband pissing, and had felt like sucking his cock clean for him when he'd finished, drinking the last drops. She hadn't dared to ask him, though, because he was far too straitlaced. He would have thought she was some kind of pervert."

Very little serious study has been made into the erotic pleasures of urination, in spite of the fact that so many men and women find it exciting and alluring. One of the principal reasons for its erotic attraction is that it represents a spectacular outpouring of fluid which can be seen as a kind of climactic ejaculation to the nth power. If only a man could shoot out so much sperm, or a woman produce so much vaginal juice!

Another reason for its attraction is its smell and its taste. Although we are highly sophisticated creatures, we still respond to strong, animal aromas, particularly those aromas associated with our sexual parts. One Denver homemaker told me that whenever her husband was away from her, she kept a pair of his dirty shorts under the pillow, so that she could breathe in the smell of his urine while she masturbated. There is an entire mail-order trade in women's "soiled panties," and a customer can even specify what sort of soiling he prefers.

But in my opinion the overwhelming reason why so many men and women derive so much pleasure from wet sex is that they feel completely liberated when they do it, both physically and emotionally. When you were very young, one of the first disciplines that your parents imposed on you was that you should urinate privately and continently. If you failed to do so you were told that you were "dirty." But if you urinate freely in front of your sexual partner, you will be casting aside one of your strictest inhibitions and sharing yourself completely. If your partner enjoys participating in that freedom by playing with your urine and urinating over you in return, then nothing is done but good. There is nothing perverted or "dirty" about it, even if you don't personally happen to like it. It's simply sex play.

Many single people also derive a high degree of erotic pleasure from self-administered enemas. I have received several letters from women who enjoy the sexual tension of filling their rectums with warm water, and holding it inside them while they masturbate. When they reach orgasm, they pull out the douche and intensify their pleasure by spurting water from their anus.

There is nothing wrong in any type of sexual self-stimulation, as long as it isn't physically dangerous. I was asked recently by a great friend of mine, a Catholic priest, "How can you possibly condone masturbation? It's completely unnatural."

But the fact is, it's *not* unnatural. Whatever the Old Testament says about poor old Onan spilling his seed on the ground, masturbation is a simple and harmless sexual pleasure, which anybody can enjoy at almost any time. Better to masturbate than to involve oneself in a fraught and complicated sexual relationship, simply for the purpose of "getting your rocks off." Better to masturbate than to feel tense and edgy and frustrated. Better to masturbate than to understand nothing at all about the way that your body responds to erotic stimulation, except what you've picked up through trial and error.

If more single women were to accept that masturbation is a perfectly acceptable way of releasing their sexual frustrations before, after, or in between lovers, perhaps more single women would avoid making rash decisions when it comes to choosing the man in their life. Sandra, 31, a tree surgeon from Madison, Wisconsin, told me: "I never masturbated all my life, never, and none of my friends did, either—unless they kept it very, very quiet. I met Steve when I was two weeks off my 21st birthday, and he had the kind of looks that turned me on *immediately*, like a switch! We were married within a month. We spent two weeks in a trailer in the woods, living off barbeque ribs and cheap champagne. It was idyllic. But although it was idyllic, I knew from day one that this wasn't it, this wasn't the sexual relationship that I'd been looking for. To cut a long story short, Steve was crude and brutal in bed, and if I didn't like what he did to me, or the way that he did it, he used to hit me. Then he used to turn me over, face down, and pull down my tights and fuck me, whether I felt like fucking or not.

"I started to masturbate when I stayed at a refuge for battered women. I think I did it for consolation to begin with. I'd lost a lot in my life. My mom died when I was ten, my pa was never well; the year before last my best friend Liz was knocked down and killed when she was crossing the street in Milwaukee. Then there was Steve.

"One of the other women at the refuge told me that her husband had caught her 'diddling,' and beaten her so badly that she hadn't been able to walk. But she said she went on doing it just the same. She didn't smoke, she didn't drink. She couldn't afford it. But she found all of the escape she needed in masturbation. 'In that split-second of having an orgasm,' she said, 'I don't have to think about anybody or anything else, only *me*."

Of course, one reason why men don't like their women to "diddle" behind their backs is because no man likes to think that his lovemaking technique may be lacking, and that the woman in his life needs to "diddle" to keep herself from going crazy. If a woman masturbates, even though she's married, or carrying on a hot 'n' heavy affair, the man in her life will immediately jump to the conclusion that he isn't keeping her satisfied.

Sometimes, of course, he may be right. But mostly, he won't be. We interviewed a sample of 300 girls between the ages of 16 and 24, and over 74 percent admitted that they had not only masturbated in between lovers, but *continued* to masturbate with only slightly less frequency during sexual relationships which were "completely fulfilling." In other words, masturbation can relieve sexual tension and reduce some of the sexual urgency that a woman may be feeling when she doesn't have a man. It's worth considering for those benefits alone.

But the real benefit of masturbation is that it teaches you about your own sexual responses, and while you're doing it, it gives you a completely private and internalized moment to consider your own sexual needs and your own sexual fantasies. It's selfish, in the very best sense of the word.

Finally—while talking to all of the women who contributed to these chapters—I conducted a survey on their favorite methods of masturbation, and drew up a Top Ten of popular masturbatory techniques:

1. Light clitoral stroking
2. Clitoral stroking plus stroking or pulling of vaginal lips
3. Rhythmical squeezing of thighs together, plus some light clitoral stimulation
4. Vaginal insertion of dildo or vibrator, plus some light clitoral stroking
5. Playing of shower on clitoral and vaginal area, plus clitoral massage
6. Breast and nipple stimulation, plus some clitoral stroking
7. Anal insertion of dildo or vibrator, plus massage of clitoris and vulva
8. Double insertion of dildoes or vibrators (vaginal and anal)
9. Sliding silk scarf backward and forward between lips of vulva
10. Vaginal insertion of any phallic object (hairbrush handle, carrot, cucumber, shampoo bottle, soda bottle, pastry pin—even, in one case, a huge sausage, liberally lubricated with KY)

SEVEN

There Must Be 900 Ways to Find a Lover

How does a single woman find a lover?

Obviously it's not nearly so difficult for *younger* single women: They're usually unhampered by children or other family ties. Not only that, they're usually part of a social circle which includes equally young and equally unattached men, such as school or college friends, or those casual groups of young people who meet in shopping malls or bowling alleys or fast-food restaurants.

Of course, there may be very good reasons why a young single woman *does* have difficulty in finding a partner. Maybe she's shy. Maybe she finds it hard to form new relationships. It could be that she's worried about committing herself, or that she's anxious about the sexual side of things. But at least there are plenty of eligible young men around—and that gives her much more of an opportunity than her older counterpart to find a potential lover, even if she has some social or sexual anxieties to overcome first.

As far as shyness is concerned, I've talked to a whole range of people about it, from clinical psychiatrists to the beauty editors of women's magazines. The consensus of opinion seems to be that the best way to deal with shyness is the old-fashioned way: to make sure that you're completely confident about the way you're dressed and the way you're groomed, and then to try as hard as you can to act proudly and speak to men with as much confidence and self-assurance as you can muster.

Never run yourself down. If a man compliments you, accept his compliment at face value and thank him for it. Never be afraid to be yourself. Everybody is interesting in their own way. And everybody is sexually attractive to *somebody,* even if you don't think that you are.

I have college-age sons of my own, and I have seen how positively they respond to girls with a bright, upbeat personality, even if those girls aren't classically "pretty" or outstandingly clever.

Of course it takes tremendous effort of will for a quiet, diffident girl to speak her mind in the company of a boy she happens to like. I'm not pretending it's easy—especially at first.

But remember that men of all ages always have at least one major recreational interest in their lives, whether it's baseball or fishing or rock music or automobiles. You can easily find out what a young man's principal interest is just by asking him a few pertinent questions. Then all you have to do is listen and ask him more questions. He'll soon wind up thinking that you're someone *very* special.

You may find that his pet interest is pretty boring (at least, to you). In that case, you're going to have to decide whether you like him enough to put up with a few hours' intense discussion about drag racing or heavy rock music or the World Series. But it really is extraordinary how warmly men respond to being asked questions about themselves—and it really is extraordinary how rarely women do it.

When you meet a man you like, think of yourself as a TV interviewer—as a Barbara Walters or an Oprah Winfrey—and you'll be astonished how easily and effectively you manage to catch his attention. Asking men questions about themselves is the quickest way to their hearts, believe me.

Beyond the small-talk, you will soon begin to discover the man himself, and when he's finished talking sports, you will frequently find that he's more than interested in talking about togetherness.

As far as sex is concerned, it really is absolutely essential to make sure that you know all about the birds and the bees and how your body works. If you have read any of my books, such as *How to Drive Your Man Wild in Bed* or *Wild in Bed Together* or *Sex Secrets of the Other Woman*, you will already have a very clear and comprehensive understanding of your sexual responses.

But *please* make sure that you have a sound knowledge of sex and sexual technique before you enter into any physically intimate relationship. And in particular, *please* make sure that you protect yourself from unwanted pregnancy and sexually communicated diseases. There are no ifs or buts about this requirement. There's nothing grown-up about giving birth to an unwanted baby, and there's nothing glamorous about contracting AIDS. Both lead to anguish, tragedy and damaged lives.

So many single women still have only the sketchiest idea about sex and sexual technique.

- "I spent all evening at a party with a man I really liked. In fact, I liked him so much that I was going to go to bed with him. When I went to the bathroom, however, I found that my vagina was wet and that my panties were soaked. I was too embarrassed to let him discover that I had wet panties, and so I made an excuse and asked him to drive me home."
- "I never seem to get any enjoyment out of sex. Most of my boyfriends have finished even before

I've gotten started. I find sex so frustrating that I feel like giving it up altogether. Don't tell me to try masturbation because I do it all the time: It's the only way I can stay sane."

- "Whenever my boyfriend makes love to me, I have fantasies that we are having sex in front of an audience. It excites me a whole lot, but I don't want to tell him about it in case he gets angry. He's one of those real jealous types."

- "Just before my period I can't think about anything but sex. I still feel ultra-horny when I'm actually having my period. Is this abnormal? I need sex so much during that time of the month but my lover always acts 'the gentleman' and doesn't touch me. Yet as soon as my period has finished, I don't feel like sex nearly so much."

These are all typical excerpts from scores of letters that have been sent to me by anxious women in the past six months. The answers to all of their questions were very straightforward, and none of my correspondents needed to be seriously worried. But it plainly would have helped their confidence if they had already been much more *au fait* with their own sexuality (both physical and emotional) *before* they entered into an intimate relationship.

- The woman who was worried about vaginal wetness had nothing to all to worry about. In fact, she should have been pleased that her physiological response to a man who attracted her was so positive. Many women have trouble with vaginal dryness, particularly in middle age. Although they can usually overcome their difficulty with hormone treatment or vaginal lubricants (of which there are a great number freely available in drugstores), they would be only too happy to have this girl's "wet panty" problem. Men's reaction to vaginal wetness is almost always one of appreciation and excitement. It is tangible proof that a woman finds them sexually attractive and that her body is preparing itself for sexual stimulation and intercourse.

- The woman who "never seemed to get any enjoyment out of sex" was a classic victim of what sexologists often call "the arousal gap"—that is, the troublesome fact that it usually takes women much longer than men to reach the same state of high sexual arousal. Young men in particular are prone to ejaculating very quickly, and so they may often have climaxed and finished while their partner is still in the very early stages of building herself up toward an orgasm. Women vary considerably in their sexual sensitivity, and some women (although they are very loving and highly sensual) need considerably more stimulation than others. There can be psychological reasons for this. For instance, she may feel inhibited about making love, or she may be worried about becoming pregnant. However, there may be physiological reasons for it, too. Every woman's clitoris is endowed with a certain number of highly responsive nerve fibers, which carry pleasure signals to the brain. Among these fibers are miniscule structures called Pacinian corpuscles, which are highly sensitive to pressure. Some women have a wealth of these corpuscles; others have fewer, which may account for the fact that some women need strong, determined stimulation to bring them to orgasm while others need only the lightest of touches. Some women, in fact, cannot bear to have the glans of their clitoris massaged directly, while others adore a strong, persistent rubbing. The way to close the "arousal gap" is to encourage your lover to indulge in more foreplay before he actually penetrates you. One of the best ways to do this is to give him oral sex, sucking and kissing his penis, while at the same time maneuvering yourself into the classic "69" position, with your vulva close to his face, so that he will be more than tempted to kiss and touch your vagina, and give you that extra stimulation you require in order to reach orgasm.

- The woman who had daydreams about making love in front of other people was expressing one of the most common of erotic fantasies, and she had absolutely no cause for concern whatsoever. One of the qualities that makes sex so exciting is its "naughtiness," its "rudeness," and its sense that you are doing something forbidden. One of the strongest taboos about sex is that you should do it in private—that is why the fantasy of doing it in front of an audience is so potent. As I have said many times before, a fantasy is only a fantasy, and you should relax and enjoy it, no matter how shocking it would be if you acted it out in real life.

- The woman who was concerned about the strength of her sexual desire during her period had very little to worry about, either. Immediately prior to menstruation, many women find that their sexual appetite increases dramatically, and they feel like making love every hour of the day. This sexual voraciousness can last all through their period, but once they actually start bleeding, intercourse can become a messy and rather off-putting procedure. Apart from that, many women report that they lose a great deal of vaginal slipperiness when they're actually menstruating, and it's quite true that rapidly drying menstrual blood can interfere with the normal friction of the erect penis inside the vagina.

The answer to "time-of-the-month" blues is to try oral or anal sex. Jackie, 23, a dental technician from Marion, Iowa, said, "James and I had only been dating for about ten days when I had a period. Up until then, everything had been going real great. We loved each other and I knew that I wanted him—well, *wanted* him, if you understand what I mean. I didn't want to lose him, ever. I wanted to walk up the aisle one day, with him wearing his full-dress Naval uniform. And I think he did, too.

"The problem was, James was real popular with all of the girls, and he only had to walk into a room and they were all clustering around him. So I was very wary about telling him that I couldn't sleep with him. He'd go off and sleep with somebody else, and they would make sure that they didn't have a period, and he'd marry her, and that would be it. My whole life in ruins!

"I talked to an older woman I know—Mary, she's 26, and she's been married for nearly four years. She said, 'You can always do it the other way.' I said, 'What do you mean, "the other way?"' And so she said, 'You can always let him make love to you up the ass.' Well, I was shocked, at first. I knew that homosexuals did it, but I never realized that men and women could do it. But Mary was really helpful and understanding. She said that her husband had encouraged her to do it when they were first married, and that she'd grown to accept it as a perfectly natural thing for a man and his wife to do together.

"So I did everything she told me. I bought some KY jelly, and I practiced by lubricating my asshole with it, and sliding things up there—only my finger at first, but then two fingers, and then a cucumber. I made the mistake of using the cucumber right out of the icebox, and *boy* was that cold! After two or three days, I realized that I *could* take something as big as James's erect cock up my asshole.

"I was out with James at Huckleberry's when it came to my period time. I was searching in my purse for some more money when James saw that I had a pack of tampons in it, along with all the makeup and the usual mess. He nodded toward them and said, 'I guess we'll have to take a raincheck tonight.' I said, 'Of course we won't. There are plenty of other things that we can do.'

"We went back to his parents' house that night. I kissed him and unbuttoned his shirt, and gently scratched him with my fingernails, all over his back and his chest. I kissed his nipples, and bit them, too, and by that time he was getting pretty turned on. I held his cock through his pants, and he was totally hard, like an iron bar.

"I knelt down in front of him, and opened his pants, and took out his cock. It was huge. I'd never felt it so stiff before. The head of his cock was deep wine red, and there was shiny juice dripping out of the opening. I cupped my hand inside his shorts, and started to lightly massage his balls. They were all wrinkled and tight. Then I licked the head of his cock, and probed into his juicy hole with the tip of my tongue, so that I could taste his juice. It was delicious. It was slippery and slightly sweet. I took the whole of his cock head in my mouth and gently sucked it. It filled my mouth right up. I loved it. I wished that I could take his whole cock into my mouth, but it was far too big. I held his cock in my hand and massaged it against my face, rubbing it against my lips and giving his cock hole little butterfly kisses with my eyelashes. Then I ran my tongue all the way down his cock to his balls, and licked all around his balls until he was moaning, and running his fingers through my hair.

"I pulled his pants right down to his ankles, and at the same time I went on licking and sucking his balls, and massaging his cock against my face.

"Then I said he should lie back on the floor, which he did. I opened my purse, and took out a mint-fragranced condom. I tore open the wrapper, pinched the little teat at the end, so that the air wouldn't get in, and unrolled it over his cock. Then I took the head of his cock into my mouth again, and gave him six or seven hard sucks, and played with the dangling teat of the condom with my tongue.

"He was going crazy! And I was incredibly turned on, too, because I'd never had so much power in any sexual relationship before. I was calling the shots. I was doing what *I* wanted to do.

"I was wearing this short thin dress of silvery-gray knitted cotton, with a gold chain belt. I lifted it up, and James saw that I wasn't wearing any panties, I was naked underneath. Not only that, but I'd shaved my pussy, so that it was completely hairless. That was Mary's idea—she said that it always drove men crazy when you shaved your pussy. I thought it looked pretty bald—you could see my clitoris and my lips and everything. Of course you could see my tampon string, too, but that didn't turn James off at all.

"He said, 'Come on, I don't mind, you can take that thing out and fuck me, can't you?' But I told him no, my period was too heavy. So he said, 'What did you put that goddamned condom on for, if you're not going to let me fuck you?' I said he could fuck me if he wanted to. I turned my back on him, and lifted up my bare bottom. Then I squeezed out a whole handful of KY jelly, and reached behind me, and smeared it all around my asshole. I think he began to get the message!

I hunkered down over his hips, with my back to him. I took hold of his cock, and it was all hard and minty-smelling. I heard him say something like "Oh, God . . ." then I positioned the head of his cock right up against my asshole, and forced my asshole open the way that Mary had told me, and sat on his huge great cock.

"I felt it slide all hot and rubbery right up inside my ass. My ass muscles kept wincing, and gripping it extra-tight, and I didn't know whether I wanted to drag it into me further or to push it right out again. He was right up my ass, his whole cock, right up to his balls, and I could feel his pubic hair against my asshole.

"I rode slowly up and down, so that his cock slid in and out of my asshole very luxuriously. I reached down and felt where we joined, James's huge slippery con-domed cock, and my stretched-open asshole. James was gripping my thighs and panting, because it took so much effort for him to thrust his cock right up inside my asshole, and because he was so turned on.

"I loved it, though. I suddenly felt free. I could make love during a heavy period. I could turn on a man like James without any trouble at all. And although it had hurt just a little to start with, I loved being fucked up the ass. I could have done it all day, it felt so good. This huge warm cock sliding in and out of my bottom! I reached behind me, and pulled my bottom cheeks apart even wider, and sat down harder and harder on James's cock, because I wanted it further and further up my ass.

"James suddenly drove himself deep inside me, and shuddered, and gasped, and I knew that he was com-ing. I reached down between my legs and held his con-dom tight around the base of his cock, in case it slipped off. Then I eased myself off him, and his cock slipped out of my asshole.

"He lay back on the rug, covered in sweat, his chest heaving up and down. I took the greatest of pleasure in pulling off his condom, and emptying out all that warm jellyish sperm, all over his cock and his balls and his stomach.

"Then I knelt right over his face, and very gently

lowered my bare-shaved pussy over his mouth, like somebody kissing somebody, mouth to mouth. I took hold of his hand, and guided it between the cheeks of my ass, so that he could feel how much my asshole had opened and swollen. It was sore, but I loved him touching it and stroking it and poking his fingers up inside it.

"We've stayed together, James and me, and we're more married than people who are married. He hasn't put on that Naval uniform yet and walked me up the aisle—but he will, he will!

"We always have anal sex when I'm going through my period, and sometimes we have it when I'm *not* going through my period. I love it; it's like having two pussies instead of one. I was worried about hygiene to begin with, but you can use a fragranced condom or a fragranced lubricant, and it's very rarely dirty. Sometimes I find myself wishing that I had two men instead of one—one up each hole, and their balls joggling together! I would recommend anal sex to any woman, provided she wants to do it, that is; and provided she's careful about contraception.

"You did ask about far-out sex, too, didn't you? Well [embarrassed] there's a thing that we do when we're really feeling naughty and dirty. Maybe I shouldn't tell you. I don't know. James—what do you think? [James shrugs, nods okay, and Jackie continues.] The thing is, we warm up the tub by filling it with hot water. Then we empty it out again. When it's empty, I climb into the tub and James follows close behind me. He lifts up the tail of my nightshirt, and exposes my bottom. Then he takes some KY and starts rubbing it around my anus. Then he kneels behind me, and pushes his bare cock into my bottom, as far as he can.

"We have to wait for a moment, because he's so turned on he can't do it instantly. But, he's made quite sure that he's drunk three or four pints of water about an hour before, and so it *does* come eventually. I can feel the hot gush of it right up inside me. He pisses up inside my ass, fills it, I can feel it. Sometimes it spurts out from between my legs, out of the sides of my asshole, even thought it's stoppered up by James's cock.

"As soon as he takes out his cock, my asshole contracts, and I think that everything's fine. I can feel his piss trickling down the backs of my thighs; and what he does then is to start fingering my clitoris, fingering it around and around the way I really love it, soft then not so soft. After only a few seconds, my bottom starts to twitch, and then suddenly his piss spurts out of my asshole, three or four long hot streams of it. That's when he kneels up behind me again, and starts to fuck me, quick and hard, and it doesn't often take him long to come. I can feel that, too, his sperm up inside my ass.

"When we're all done, all we have to do is turn on the shower attachment and spray ourselves down. What can I say? I've never told anybody about this before, but not because I'm ashamed of it. How can a woman be ashamed of having the cock of the man she loves up inside her body, no matter how she does it? James respects me and loves me, and the way we make love is part of what we are: one hundred percent close, one hundred percent uninhibited. And able to have sex all the way through my period, too, just when I'm feeling my horniest."

You needn't get yourself involved in any extra anal variations such as wet sex or urine enemas if they don't excite you. But many millions of women all over the world enjoy anal intercourse as a natural alternative to vaginal sex, particularly during their monthly period. In the 1970s the New York Sex Research Foundation surveyed 3,000 men and women and found that 25 percent of all married couples had experimented with anal intercourse. And in Germany, the RALF report sent questionnaires to 10,000 men and women and had roughly the same response—22 percent of women said they had experience of anal intercourse, and 18 percent of men had, too. *The Janus Report* suggests that a third of American men and women positively approve of anal sex.

You can train yourself to enjoy a stunning degree of erotic stimulation from anal intercourse. First of all, you have to rid yourself of the idea that it's "dirty." The rectum contains little or no fecal matter until you actually need to go to the toilet. It *does* harbor millions of virulent bacteria, however, and you should always take care to wash your hands and genitals thoroughly after anal play. You should *never* allow your lover to insert his penis into your anus and then directly into your vagina. You could contract a nasty infection.

But with sensible and straightforward precautions, anal intercourse can be nothing but stimulating fun.

Learning to make love anally can take a little perseverance, not to mention a considerable amount of care and sensitivity on the part of your lover. You won't always feel like doing it (and if you *don't* feel like doing it, you are quite entitled to say "no." It's your body, after all). But a surprisingly high proportion of the women I have talked to about sexual technique say that "with the right man, with a man you really love, anal intercourse can open out all kinds of fantastic new feelings, all kinds of new possibilities. It's emotional as well as physical. When a man thrusts his penis into your bottom, you really feel as if you're being *taken*. Not like rape, but taken because you want to be taken."

We've looked at some of the problems that worry a young single woman when she's trying to establish an intimate relationship with a man. But older single women who are looking for a lover face a much more difficult problem. They may be more sexually experienced and know much more about lovemaking techniques, but where are the men for them to practice on?

More often than not, older women are single because they're divorced or separated, or because they've been involved in a long-term relationship that hasn't, in the end, been as long-term as they had expected.

In the United States, the average age of bridegrooms is 28, so it doesn't take a demographic genius to work out that a divorced woman of 29 is going to find herself all on her own in a world in which a large percentage of the most eligible men are already partnered off. In other words, her sexual options have been drastically reduced.

These days, a woman of 28-plus is still very young. A woman of 38-plus is still young. And women in their mid-forties are still so sexually attractive that there is even a sexy magazine published in Germany called *Uber 40,* showing mature women in nothing but pearl necklaces and black basques, with their legs wide apart. But if a woman over 28 suddenly finds herself single, she has to face the bitter, bitter truth that far too many of those handsome young bucks of her school and college days have gone and gotten themselves married.

"My husband and I parted because we simply didn't love each other any longer," said Caroline, a 36-year-old journalist from Washington, D.C. "We just woke up one morning and stared at each other and said, 'That's it, it's over.'

"We're still friends. We'll probably stay friends till one of us dies. But I couldn't see the point of staying with a man just because I kind of like him. Mind you, there were plenty of times in the months to come when I wish I *had* stayed with him, just for the comfort and the companionship.

"Alan moved out and found a small house in Silver

Spring. I was left with a large apartment and Jonas, our eight-year-old son, and two cats. I work from home so there was no real difficulty with daytime baby-sitters or anything like that, which was a blessing, I suppose. But all the same, I found that Jonas *was* a tie. I couldn't decide to stay out all night whenever I felt like it. I couldn't spend a weekend by the seashore at the drop of a hat. And men definitely found it off-putting when I told them that I had a son. That meant that if they were ever going to get serious with me—I mean *really* serious, like becoming my husband—they were going to have to think about being a stepfather to Jonas, too.

"Well, to begin with, I couldn't find any men at all, let alone any men who wanted to be my husband. I had never realized how difficult it is for a single, mature woman to find herself a partner. When Alan and I were together, we were invited out regularly—two or three times a week, sometimes more often. There were always parties and cookouts and theater evenings and charity events. Suddenly I found that I wasn't being invited to anything anymore, except the occasional all-girls-together coffee-morning or wedding shower. I told my friends that Alan and I were getting divorced, but I might just as well have said, 'I have leprosy.'

"Within the space of only a few weeks, my entire life was changed beyond recognition. I felt so much better for having broken up with Alan—emotionally, I mean. I felt so much freer, so much more able to be myself. There were so many unrealized things in my life that I wanted to do. Paint, read, *think*. It's so hard to find time to *think* when you're married—especially when you're married to a man as talkative and as opinionated as Alan.

"Suddenly I discovered that I had my own views about politics, and music, and food, and wine. I stopped drinking Orvieto and started drinking California chardonnay. I stopped eating red meat. Even though I was stressed out, especially during the divorce itself, I found that I didn't actually like smoking, and I stopped doing that, too.

"The problem was, I was hardly ever invited to any dinner parties where I might meet an eligible man. When I *was* invited, I usually found that I had been partnered with a man who was *very* much older than me and whose social deficiencies were glaringly obvious (like a toupee, or halitosis, or an enlarged prostate). Either that, or they were handsome as hell and just the right age and witty and charming and gay. And quite often angry because they had been matched with *me* and not their own partner."

I have heard this anguished story so many times. For an older woman, the pain of separation is followed by the greater and far more long-lasting pain of finding somebody to love her. And the sadness is that so many women of 28-plus are in the full bloom of their beauty and their sexuality. They are bold, engaging, and experienced lovers, and they are quite capable of giving any man the sexual time of his life.

But where are the men who would so much enjoy their sexual favors, and where does a single woman go to find them?

Journalist Lesley Garner was recently divorced from her husband. She said: "In a world full of single women I have had many conversations with women friends who are baffled about the whereabouts of the other half. Of course, many men rush on to younger second wives. Men are also less brave about being left alone than women—many line up their next relationship before they leave the coziness of the first. But that still leaves thousands unaccounted for."

She decided that, on the whole, they were "in hiding," too stoical or cowardly to take a second chance.

"Maybe they are right to avoid women because women are largely on the hunt for a new partner."

Financial anxieties also inhibit men from forming new relationships, particularly if they still have a first family to support. They shy away from the thought of a permanent situation because they are apprehensive about the cost of maintaining a second woman. One man, celibate for 10 years, said that he relished the freedom of long walks in the hills on his own. Not that he wasn't interested in sex, but "the emotional rollercoaster of sexual passion scares me, rather than excites me, as I get further into middle age."

It's interesting to find out, however, that even in celibate hill-walkers, the passion is still there somewhere. A woman kissed our hero at an office party, and he said, " 'I haven't been swamped by a mass of perfumed hair and the taste of lipstick for 10 years. So you don't need to really fall in love or go to bed with someone to suffer from 'agony and ecstasy.' "

Lesley Garner concluded: "If the women could expect less and the men become a little braver, the sun of affectionate companionship might shine."

From the previous two chapters, we have seen that a great many single people—both men and women—satisfy their immediate sexual urges by masturbating. Men also have the option of visiting prostitutes or massage parlors for "full relief," or any number of sexual services in between. A recent issue of a men's magazine offered: "Dirty Letter Club—write dirty letters to our female members and receive dirty letters from our female/gay/AC-DC members." It also offered telephone services that varied from "Suzie Uses a Sausage" to "Cum All Over Me" and "Let me lick your balls, baby, I'll make you shoot!" Then there are offers from: "Gail, elegant blonde, gives special unhurried massage" and "Two young Swedish female students (just 18) touring

US want free bed and breakfast on their travels. Willing to pay in kind."

Unfortunately, women's magazines rarely feature the same kind of sexual services. This isn't because women wouldn't respond to such services if they were offered. Women are just as intent on seeking sexual satisfaction as men, if not more so. The problem is that we live in a male-dominated society that tolerates the use of call girls or massage parlors by frustrated husbands, but seriously frowns on rent boys or massage parlors for women.

Gail, 39, a beautiful blonde from San Francisco, said: "I keep seeing these massage ads in the papers, and I'd *love* to have a sexual massage. I have a fantasy about lying back on a massage table while an elegant young Chinese man rubs oil into my body and then slides his fingers between my buttocks, and just 'peeps' his fingertip into my cunt. I pretend that I'm sleeping, and so he grows bolder, and slides his finger into my cunt, all the way up to the knuckle, and starts stroking my clitoris, too. I still pretend that I'm sleeping, and so he slides another finger into my ass, and starts to massage my cunt and my ass with this wonderful round-and-round wriggling with his fingers. I have a deep, deep orgasm, but I really suppress it. He pretends that he hasn't noticed. It's like some kind of unspoken etiquette. Afterward, I pay him and leave, and that's all there is to it. I love that fantasy. I love the sexual tension of it. I love all the unspoken sexuality. It makes me wet myself just thinking about it. My panties are wet now, just *talking* about it. If I could find a massage parlor that could recreate that fantasy for me, for real, then I'd be there, in 15 minutes flat, with my credit card ready."

Gail was sexually disadvantaged just because she was a woman. There are scarcely any commercial facilities that offer sexual services for women. Of course there *are* massage parlors for women, but most of them are legitimate beauty establishments, and very few will provide sexual relief. There are thousands of male prostitutes, too, but the pressures of street economics means that the majority of them are homosexuals or bisexuals, and the risks of contracting the HIV virus from a casually picked-up man are far too high to be seriously entertained.

Not only that, a male prostitute may well have a drug problem, and young men with drug problems can be unpredictably violent and prone to theft or even worse. It's my advice that you should catch yourself a live lover, fresh out of the water. And you should set your sights very high indeed.

Paid-for sex has none of the wild, deep eroticism that you're really looking for. Neither has casual sex—the kind of sex that Erica Jong described as "the zipless fuck." You might enjoy a quick stand-up fuck in back of the office; or a thrusting few minutes in an airplane washroom, at 36,000 feet. But at your age, and with your experience, you're capable of giving your heart and giving your soul, so why settle for anything less? You want to be where the wild things are, don't you?

You've been masturbating, to keep those sexual urges in check. But you're interested in finding a truly exciting sexual relationship, and so (all in good time) you're looking for more than dildo-induced orgasms and hand-aroused climaxes. There's nothing wrong in either form of sexual stimulation—or, indeed, *any* form of sexual stimulation that makes you feel better and isn't physically or psychologically harmful. But a wild and exciting sex life demands more than self-stimulated climaxes (or even "full relief massage," as pleasurable as that "full relief" may be).

A wild and exciting sex life starts with shared emotion and shared commitment. It needs both tenderness and strength. It cries out for surrender. At the same time it demands domination. More than anything else, it requires total openness, body and soul, by *both* of you.

These are qualities that you can only find with a partner whom you can respect and care for, and (sooner or later) learn to love. These are qualities that take time to find, and that require patience, tact, dedication, and, above all, a high degree of sexual self-esteem. You are a woman and you are beautiful. You deserve the best. But you will only *get* the best if you expect the best.

So, if you don't go out and buy your sexual satisfaction on the street, like many lonely men do, where *do* you look for it?

You can try some of the more respectable-looking singles bars. You can try social clubs or the dinner-party circuit, with an occasional foray into Sunday brunches and cocktail parties and vacation-time cookouts. Yes, I know. All of these may seem like pretty tame places to meet a man, especially when you compare them with glitter and the glitz of big-city vice. But these days, safety has to be regarded as one of the most important priorities in meeting men and women for "intimate relationship—love—possibly marriage.'

You will find a page of advice at the end of this book that will help to protect you against AIDS. But you will also need to use your common-sense to protect yourself against confidence tricksters, time wasters, and men who suddenly turn violent for no apparent reason at all.

The rules are very basic, but it's amazing how many women don't even think about them when they go out on a date with a complete stranger. Before you say "yes," and agree to go, ask him the following questions: Where do you live? Where do you work? Where are you going to collect me? Where and when are you going to bring me home? What is your telephone number? (And make sure you call back with another question, no matter how fatuous—like "Would you like to see me in duck-egg blue or emerald green?" That way, you'll know for sure that his number is legitimate.)

When you go out on that date, tell a trusted friend where you're going and when you expect to be back. (If you're planning on going to bed with your date, don't be embarrassed about saying "tomorrow morning.") And make sure your trusted friend knows the details of your date's automobile—make, model, color, and license.

All of this may sound like paranoia, especially when a good-looking man has just asked you out on a date and all *you* feel like is candlelight and music and the wind in your hair. But take a few moments to take sensible precautions, and you'll never regret it. Particularly if you emphasize now and again that you have friends who care for you and who know where you are ("Jane was so jealous when I told her you were taking me to Oscar's for dinner").

Many single women will now be asking me: How do I get that date in the first place? I'd do anything for any man to take me anyplace at all, let alone some suave hunk taking me to Oscar's.

The answer is: You should try the personals.

The personals! So many women have said to me, despairingly, "I'd rather die than look for a man in the personals."

But these days, the personals make a whole lot of sense. There's nothing sad or defeatist about them. How can it be any more demeaning to meet a lover through a personal than it is to meet him at a party or a dance or a church barbecue? In fact, the personals are not demeaning in the slightest. They give lonesome people an opportunity to meet other lonesome people, that's all. And why should it be any more humiliating to answer a man's advertisement in a magazine than to talk to him face-to-face at a neighborhood cookout? If he wants companionship, and *you* want companionship, and you both like each other, what's the problem?

Many women said, "Men tell so many lies in their personal ads. How can I trust them?" My answer to that is: Men always tell lies anyway, and so do women. We always want to present ourselves in the best possible light. That's an integral part of the game of flirting. All you have to do is to use your common sense and interpret the personals in the most literal way possible. "Fun-loving" means flippant, with a short attention span, and unwilling to discuss anything more serious than where to go for dinner. "Travels a lot" means married. "Absolutely unique" means a nervy, eccentric, argumentative person who has never been able to get along with anybody. If a man says he's "huggable" or a woman says she's "Rubenesque," then they're fat.

Here's an interpretative list of personal adjectives. I don't mean my interpretations to be derogatory, but I've answered all of the personals carrying these descriptions, and tried to reconcile the printed come-on with the reality.

- "Intense DWM"—divorced man still carrying an oxyacetylene torch for his first wife, looking for an understanding woman to support him in his ferocious tussles against her . . . a woman whom he can flaunt in front of his ex-wife to make her feel jealous . . . and a woman whom he will drop like a hot potato if there is any chance of going back.
- "Vibrant intelligent passionate SWM"—overopinionated and overeducated thirtysomething with views about everything, looking for yet another woman to put through his meat-mincer of liberal dogma. To begin with, he will make love night and day, but his ardor will rapidly cool when he begins

to lose interest, and he will go back to saving the seals.

- "Gentle whimsical male physician"—nutty, narrow-minded doctor who always jogs at exactly the same time every day, who listens to the same three Beethoven symphonies over and over, who likes appallingly pretentious restaurants where they bring you the check in an antique book. Also keen on black lacy underwear and women who wear high heels in bed. He will never be able to carry on a stable long-term sex relationship because his beeper is always beeping.
- "Ocean-loving DWM"—his first wife left him because he was always messing around with his yacht, and he will now expect you to do the same. Don't answer unless you're prepared to be a second mate in every sense of the word.
- "Fit, active professional DWM"—divorced man who has become obsessed with his own health. He jogs, he cycles, he scuba dives, you name it. He will also give you backrubs and foot massages from hell. He will only ever love one person: himself.
- "Quiet fortysomething SWM"—lonesome depressive, no matter what he says in his personal. He will ask for "any woman between 20 and 40," which really means that he will accept a woman over 23 if he's forced to, but only just.
- "Woody Allen type"—he has the Woody Allen fashion sense, the Woody Allen physique, and the Woody Allen penchant of never shutting up. Unfortunately he doesn't have the Woody Allen wit.

This list isn't meant to put you off. I have included it simply to make you aware that the personals can be brilliantly worthwhile when you find the person you really want, but you *do* have to be well prepared for jokers and failures and men you half-like but not enough to go to bed with them.

Look for the plain, heartfelt message. Look for the straight statement and the unexpected declaration of honesty. "I'm not a genius, but . . ." "Nobody has ever mistaken me for Warren Beatty, but . . ." Look for the minimal ads—the ads that tell you, plain and simple, that a man is looking for love.

When it comes down to basics, very few women who read the personals are looking for men with academic or professional credentials, and even fewer are looking for men with impressive incomes or acres of real estate or prestigious job status. The Porsches don't appeal; the fine wines don't fascinate. Women who play the personals are looking for men who are friendly, warm, and emotionally accessible. They are looking for men who are not afraid to give their hearts to them deeply and without reservation, and who are able to be loved back in equally generous measure. Even if he drives an '81 Caprice and wears tweed coats from J. C. Penney, they're looking for a lover.

You should never be embarrassed about playing the personals. Maybe your safely married friends will lift some eyebrows. But the very best of single people are using them today. In fact, personals are one of the most effective social media ever, because they give you the chance to meet equally lonesome men in distant cities, men who are desperately keen for a loving relationship but whom you would never normally meet.

These days, personals appear in all kinds of magazines and newspapers—from city magazines like *Boston* and *Los Angeles* to your local *Pennysaver*. Even *The Washington Post* has started to accept personals.

The greatest boost to the personals boom has been the introduction of voice mail. Almost all personals now carry a 900 number. If you like the description in the advertisement, you can call the 900 number and listen to a prerecorded message from the advertiser. If you're still intrigued, you can leave a message.

The 900-number calls are routed for more than 100 alternative newspapers all across the country by Tele-Publishing Inc. of Boston, and at the time of writing they were dealing with more than 150,000 calls a week (and rising). There are similar services in Britain and several other countries in Europe.

You would think in the age of AIDS, when single women think that they should be able to examine a man's entire medical history before sharing a box of popcorn with him, that personals would have declined. Instead, they're burgeoning, and there are several very good reasons.

They're simple to use. They're comparatively safe. You don't have to commit yourself to a face-to-face meeting until you're totally happy about the credentials of the man you're meeting. You can listen to a voice-mail number again and again, to make absolutely certain that you like the sound of the man you're interested in, and that there aren't any sexual or psychological undertones in his message that make you feel uneasy. This is something you *can't* do at a party or a singles bar. No man is going to take it very kindly if you keep saying: "Would you mind repeating that sentence you just said about being forceful with women?"

Compared with relationships that start through chance meetings, the relationships that stem from personals have a remarkable survival rate. After all, both partners have gone deliberately looking for a particular type of lover, and both partners are usually prepared to invest a great deal of emotional effort into making sure that their new romance has everything that their old romance lacked.

Even so, many single women are still very reluctant to use personals. They regard the business of advertis-

ing for a mate to be brazen, aggressive, humiliating—
and even, so help me, "loose."

But whatever failings the people who place the personals might have, looseness, aggression, and brazen-
ness are very rarely among them. As one single woman
put it: "I liked the straightforwardness of the personals.
In the pursuit of love or the best piece of fish at the
fish store, I'm in favor of saying what you're looking
for rather than leaving it to some mind reader to figure
it out."

We advertise for automobiles, for apartments, for
daily help, for almost everything we need. There are
literally thousands of sex-line numbers, offering live
and prerecorded "turn-ons": "Jane Wants to Be Your
Sex Slave," "Trixie Has a Sex Shave," "Full Orgasmic
Groans," "I Can Take It All up Me." If we can advertise
for services like that, why should we be ashamed to
advertise for love?

Let's take a look at some of the women who found
sexual fulfillment through personal ads and voice-mail,
and at how you can script your own personal advertisement so that you can find the man you're *really* looking
for.

EIGHT

Looking for Mr. Goodsex

Cindy, a pretty brunette from Richmond, Virginia, found herself single at the age of 34 after an acrimonious divorce from her husband Tom.

"I thought that Tom and I were all settled down for a lifetime of happiness together," she told me. "But it wasn't to be. He took up with another girl and said that he'd found himself true love. I didn't think that she was anywhere near as pretty as me, and I told him so. That's when he said that I was vain and selfish, and that I never thought about nothing except how attractive I was looking.

"That remark cut me deeply. But I thought about it long and hard, and there was a lot of truth in it. I decided that I was going to try to change my attitude toward life, and that I was going to find myself a man to whom I could *prove* that I had changed."

Although most of her friends were surprised and many of them expressed strong disapproval, Cindy tried "playing the personals."

"I bought every newspaper and magazine that I could find that ran personals. I spent hours going through them. I marked all the ones that interested me with a highlighter pen, and then I narrowed them down to a short list of three. Some of them sounded really fabulous. 'Absolutely unique SWM, PhD, 43, attractive, slim, intellectual, interested in art, history, serious music, canoeing, ethnic food, Golden Retrievers. Seeks intellectual, attractive, slim, professional SF 27–35, who wants to be best friend and lover, eventual family, prefers learning/adventure vacation in Egypt or India rather than tanning in Bermuda.'

"And here's another one: 'Successful author, handsome and zestful, avid skier, seeks romantic relationship with sensual, affectionate, curvaceous creative woman.'

"And another—just listen to this one—'We are ocean spirits, lovers of sunsets, collectors of people not things. You are strikingly beautiful and youthful in age and/or spirit, the kind of woman who would complement a handsome, sailing yachtsman and successful enterpreneur/financier. Yet your beauty also comes from within. You are very caring and empathetic yet respectful of space. Outwardly respectable. But behind closed doors you are full of mischief. I am DWM, 52, blue eyes, sandy hair, full of adventure and laughter, with classic midwestern values. I am warm, honest, stable, loyal and possess an unusual blend of masculinity and sensitivity. Business success has allowed me to play when I choose. Please respond because I am "trophy quality." '

"I mean, does that man sound too good to be true, or does he sound too good to be true? And to begin with, those were the kind of personals I answered.

"That was my first mistake. Although I met one or two quite glamorous guys, they were so smooth and full of themselves that I just couldn't get along with them. I met one guy called Ted who owned a specialist automobile business not far from Richmond. He was tall and tanned and *very* handsome. He could talk about anything, too. We met for dinner and he talked about classical music and pop music and psychology and art and science and politics. His conversation was interesting and anecdotal and humorous. He amused me for *hours*. He didn't hog the conversation, either.

He asked me all about myself, and what my interests were, and he sat and listened and never interrupted.

"And that was the trouble. He never interrupted. What was more, he obviously didn't like it when *I* tried to interrupt him. He wasn't actually talking to me: he was giving me a speech. The second time I met him, I began to realize that he wasn't interested in my opinion at all: he was listening to me only because he knew that no woman would sit through a five-hour date without being allowed to get a word in edgewise. He wanted sex. He made that clear right from the very beginning, but I told him very firmly that I never went to bed with anybody on a first date, ever. He wanted a pretty woman on his arm. He took me to one of his favorite restaurants, and he really enjoyed it when the maitred' gave him a compliment on his taste in women.

"But more than having a pretty woman on his arm, and even more than sex, he wanted an audience. He was completely in love with himself—and all he wanted a woman around him for was to keep on telling him how amusing and handsome and virile and all-round wonderful he was. He was pretty cut up when I said that I didn't think there was any point in our continuing to see each other. His vanity was bruised, poor thing. He went on calling me and sending me roses for *weeks* afterward. But I never saw him again.

"I learned a lot from Ted, though, and from all of the other guys who wrote personals that were full of tropical beaches and fancy summer houses and BMWs and 'sensitive evenings in front of a blazing fireplace.' Those guys were almost always single because they had decided exactly what kind of life they wanted to lead, and they weren't going to change it in any respect for anybody. They had their car, they had their boat, they had their expensive apartment, and most of all they had their routine. There was another guy I dated called Jim. He was a psychotherapist. I'd answered his ad because he said he liked 'life in the fast lane,' and I thought I could use a little of that.

"Jim was good looking and funny and I liked him a lot. I thought, Here is somebody I could definitely go to bed with, if not think of marrying, even. That was, until he took me back to his apartment. I'd already started to grow a little suspicious about his fussy behavior because he had made me wipe my shoes on the grass before I got into his Mercedes. He didn't want mud on his honey-colored carpeting.

"He had a beautiful apartment. It was full of art and tasteful sculpture and beautiful rugs. And it was tidy. I'll tell you how tidy it was: Every CD was in alphabetical order. Every shirt in his closet was graded according to color. When we walked in, he asked me to take off my shoes and he asked me my shoe-size so that he could lend me a pair of mules. He had all sizes, all graded according to size. I started to feel paranoid right from the start. The crunch came when he showed me the bathroom. The toilet paper was folded into a point at the end, like they do it in hotels. I said, as a joke, "I hope you don't expect me to fold it up like that every time I use it. I'm not very good at origami.' He looked me right in the eye, and very seriously said, 'I would appreciate it if you did.' I had one drink and then I left. I couldn't see myself reaching orgasm with a psychotherapist who insisted on folding his toilet paper.

"The other thing I learned was that vanity is deeply unattractive—even more unattractive than I could have believed. Meeting those men cured me of my own vanity completely, and if I'm grateful to all of them for anything, it's that. They showed me that if you want to find a lover you have to *be* a lover, and being a lover means being prepared to give yourself, being prepared to take risks, being prepared to make changes in your life to accommodate the other person.

"I contacted men through voice mail who lived as

far away as Charlottesville and Roanoke Rapids and yet they wanted *me* to do all the traveling to meet them. They weren't even prepared to drive halfway. When I protested, they couldn't understand what they were supposed to have said wrong. I said if you won't drive halfway to meet me, how can I expect you to meet me halfway in a relationship? One of them got quite angry and swore at me.

"In the end, I answered an ad that said nothing more than 'DWM, 41, good-looking, seeks warm and serious relationship.' That's how I met Gary.

"Gary's a corporate lawyer. He's tall, quiet, and his ad didn't lie—he *is* good looking. We met for dinner at one of my favorite restaurants, and we simply clicked. He didn't give any speeches. He didn't try to impress me with his amazing exploits. He simply told me what kind of work he did and what kind of things he liked to do. He asked me questions that showed that he was genuinely interested in finding out about me, and he didn't mind my interrupting him.

"Occasionally, one or the other of us would stray into talking about our exes; but I didn't mind and neither did he. What interested me was that he was prepared to accept some of the blame for the breakup of his marriage. So many men tell you in sentence one that 'it was all that bitch's fault.' I blame Tom for being unfaithful, for sure, but I also blame myself for being so self-obsessed and never taking an interest in the things that were important to him. If you're never prepared to take the blame for things that go wrong in your relationships, you're going to go on making the same mistakes over and over.

"Gary didn't even try to kiss me that first night. But he took hold of my hands in both of his, and he showed me with his smile and his eyes that he really liked me. He also said, 'Can I see you again?' and when I said,

'Sure, when?' he said, 'Is tomorrow lunchtime too soon?'

"I thought about him all night. I had that tingle again, that fantastic tingle you get when you first start to fall in love. I couldn't believe it. I hadn't felt it in so long that I'd almost forgotten what it was like.

"I met Gary the next day at a quarter of twelve. We were both early. We were both so excited we were just like a couple of kids. We had a quick, light lunch and he held me my hand across the table. He said, 'I couldn't stop thinking about you all night,' and I said, 'Me neither.'

"After lunch he asked me if I would like to see where he lived. He said, 'No strings,' which gave me the option of saying no to sex if I wanted to, but we both knew what this was leading up to. I wanted him, and he wanted me, and that was all there was to it.

"He has a beautiful second-story apartment in an old nineteenth-century house in the Church Hill district. It's painted white and airy, and very prettily furnished, but it's relaxed, too. There was a ginger cat sleeping on the sofa, and that endeared me to Gary immediately: I like a man who keeps a cat.

"He poured us both a large glass of chilled white wine, and then he took me through to the bedroom to show me the balcony. We stood on the balcony overlooking the garden and it was a gorgeous warm day. It was then that he kissed me for the first time. He was a firm, strong, sensitive kisser. He sent shivers all the way down to my feet.

"He took me inside. The windows were still open, and the net curtains kept billowing all around us. We kissed some more, and then he caressed my breasts through my dress. I said, 'Do you think we're doing the right thing?' and he said, 'If this isn't right, then I have absolutely no conception of what "right" is.' I'll never forget him saying that.

"He unbuttoned my dress at the back, all the way down, and slipped it off my shoulders. I loved the sure, confident way he undressed me, even though the buttons were very tiny, and his fingers are very big. It made me feel really feminine: it made me feel as if I was in the hands of a man. My dress dropped to the floor, and I was standing in front of him in nothing but my bra and these very tiny lace panties. He said, 'I know you. You're the woman I've been looking for.'

"He picked me up, and laid me down on the bed, and kissed me. He kissed my neck and shoulders and when he kissed my ears . . . he had a way of gently biting my earlobes that made me think *ohhhhhhhh* . . . this is it! Then he unfastened my bra. He just slipped it off so that I scarcely felt it. He touched my nipples with his fingertips, and then he kissed them, and took them into his mouth, and sucked them, and flicked them with the tip of his tongue. I could feel them stiffening, right up against the roof of his mouth. Nobody had ever made me feel so sexy before, just by touching and kissing my breasts.

"He did something else, too, that really turned me on. He lifted my breasts and kissed me and licked me right underneath them, and then he took a whole mouthful of breast and gently sucked it. The feeling he gave me was absolutely sensational. I couldn't believe it. I almost felt as if I was going to have an orgasm in my breasts, if you can understand what I mean. My nipples were sticking out, and he kept on pinching them and rolling them and squeezing them between his fingers. I almost wished I could have shown him how much he was turning me on by squirting out milk. A friend of mine, Rita, she was suckled by her husband long after she stopped breastfeeding her baby, and she still gives milk whenever she has an orgasm . . . her husband adores it.

"Anyway, Gary kissed my stomach and my hips, and

he gave me the shivers. He trailed his fingers all the way down the sides of my thighs, and then he began to caress *inside* my thighs, and touch my panties.

"Most men are so keen to get inside of your panties as soon as possible, this really made a change. And it turned me on, too. He stroked the outside of my panties, and then he started to curl his fingertips into the elastic at the side. I was very excited by then. He kept kissing my thighs. Then he put his head down and licked all the way down the side of my panties, and all the way around them.

"He pushed his tongue into the side of my panties, and started licking my cunt lips, and tugging at my pubic hair with his teeth. Then he gently pulled my panties to one side, so that my cunt was completely bare. He pushed my legs apart . . . not forcefully, not like he was raping me—more like a hair stylist nudges your head when he's cutting your hair.

"He opened my cunt lips with his fingers, and he licked all the way around my cunt. I was embarrassed because I was so wet . . . all that breast fondling! But he reassured me by putting his whole mouth over my cunt, and gently sucking, and swallowing . . . which made me feel that he didn't find my cunt-juice disgusting or off-putting at all . . . in fact, he found it delicious and desirable.

"He licked my asshole. Nobody had ever done that to me before, and when he started to do it, I went all stiff, and clenched the cheeks of my bottom, and tried to stop him. But he gently eased me back on the bed, and kept on licking me there. I don't know whether I liked it at first—his tongue going around and around my asshole, and occasionally his tongue tip dipping into it—but after a while I relaxed and I began to enjoy it. I thought: It gives him pleasure to do it, why shouldn't I enjoy it, too?

"I lifted my legs, and opened them wide, so that he

could lick me as deeply as he wanted to. He licked me all around my asshole, and then he turned his attention to my cunt. He stuck his tongue right up my cunt, and gently sucked me at the same time. It was that combination of confidence and gentleness that really turned me on. He spent some time licking my pee hole, too, pushing the tip of his tongue into it, and sucking all around it. I don't know *what* I felt about that. Nobody had ever done it before. It was strange, and exciting, but was *so* strange, and *so* exciting, that I really couldn't work out whether it was sexy or irritating or neither or both.

"He worked up from there to my clitoris, and his tongue tip went around and around it—so lightly that he was scarcely touching it. I never felt so turned on in my life. It felt dangerous; it felt sexy. But all the time I felt *safe*, too, because he was making love to me so gently. He flicked his tongue on either side of my clitoris, and then down the shaft, I could actually feel him licking down the shaft.

"At the same time he slid his finger into my cunt, and stirred it around in a way that I had never felt before. He used his finger like a corkscrew, it went around and around in this beautiful kind of twisting movement, while his tongue kept flicking at my clitoris. He kept on touching and licking and stroking my cunt as if he couldn't get enough of it.

"I thought that I ought to be doing something to *him,* and I ruffled his hair and tried to reach down and scratch his back with my fingernails. But then I realized that I was turning him on simply by opening up my legs for him, and letting him lick my clitoris and finger my cunt, and that he wanted me to stay passive. Not submissive, but passive, at least while he was going down on me. He wanted to feel that he had the power to turn me on, from nothing at all to a really fantastic orgasm—that was what turned *him* on.

"So I lay back and I closed my eyes and I let Gary do it, and it was amazing. For the first time in my life I actually gave in to a man. But I wasn't really giving in. I was simply allowing myself to be seduced, allowing a man to turn me on, and enjoying it, without making a fuss about it, without turning it into a fight. I suddenly began to understand that men and women are very different, sexually—that men are excited by different things, and it's not because they don't respect women. In fact, they adore them. It's just that women don't understand that a man can suck and lick their cunt and enjoy it more than the best cordon bleu dinner they've ever had.

"Gary climbed onto the bed next to me and opened my legs even wider, and licked at my cunt and my clitoris until I thought I was going to die with the feeling of it. I could feel my hips rising, and that's always a sure sign that I'm close to coming. At least when he was kneeling next to me I could fondle his ass and his lovely heavy hairy balls, and stroke my hand up and down his cock. His cock was 100 percent rigid, bursting with veins, and there was slippery juice dripping from his cock hole and all down my arm. I rubbed him slowly up and down and he groaned like I'd hurt him, only I knew that I hadn't.

"I wriggled myself right underneath him, and licked the head of his cock, and rubbed it against my lips, all slippery and salty and hot. He tried to pull away from me, so that he could concentrate on giving *me* an orgasm first, but I wouldn't let him. I sucked and licked his cock, and fondled those gorgeous tight wrinkly balls, with their long dark silky hairs—and then I came—before I was ready, before I was expecting it, it just upped and swamped me, and spun me around, and carried me away. It was dark and it was light and it was warm and it was beautiful. I rubbed Gary's cock with both hands, and I heard him shout out. Then his warm, thick come was dropping all over me, like tropical rain. I closed my eyes and let it fall, and I hoped that it would fall forever. It fell on my forehead, it fell on my neck, it dropped in my eyes. I wiped it with my hand and smelled it, and there is no smell like it, not in the whole wide world. The smell of a man's come.

"I knew then that I had done the right thing, and made the right decision, and that sometimes it takes a leap in the dark to help you to sort out your problems—a leap of faith. I would recommend the personals to any woman who's looking for a man. It's kind of slow, yes. But it's comparatively safe, and it allows you the time to sit back and think, 'Hold on, now, is this really the guy for me?' "

If you're thinking of looking for a partner in the personal columns, there are some important pointers that you should try to remember.

1. *Define exactly what kind of man you're looking for.* Before you read a single personal ad, write yourself a full list of all the qualities that are essential for you in a lover—the qualities on which you refuse to compromise. Age? Education? Profession? Interests? Remember that some men of 55 are active and energetic, but others may be seven-eighths of the way over the hill. Remember also that some men with college degrees make no money whatsoever and may be as dull as dishwater. Don't try to hedge your bets, and don't try to be too subtle.

   If you really hate sports, you wouldn't be wise to date a baseball fanatic (and don't think you're going to like a golfer any better.) If you're bored to distraction by museums, you wouldn't be wise to date an Egyptologist. Do you want your lover to be smoking or nonsmoking? Can you tolerate social drinking or do you insist on no drinking at all? How about animals? Pets or no pets? Sailing or no sailing? Religion? (If religion isn't a critical issue, you could broaden your trawl by subscribing to some of the more selective contact magazines such as *The Jewish Professional*. Some DJMs insist on DJFs, while a great many more don't really give a damn.)

List any characteristic that could come any way close to creating a make-or-break problem. Anything that makes you totally switch off. And when you read those personals every day, *no matter how much you may be tempted*, don't compromise on any one of those essential qualities. Those are your basic criteria. Those are the standards that you are going to insist on, even if takes a few months longer for you to find Mr. 37-Year-Old Nonsmoking Teetotaller with a Refined Taste in Wines, No Byzantine Marital History, No Kids, and the Kind of Bank Balance That Makes You Swallow Your Tongue.

If your potential lover can't meet any one of the essential criteria that you have listed on your piece of paper, then don't answer his ad. Don't. You've probably had quite enough grief already. You certainly don't need more. If you try dating a man who doesn't fulfil your fundamental needs, you'll be wasting your time (and your emotions) and his too.

Make sure that you think very hard about one of the most important of all criteria, and that is location. Most professional men have built their careers in one particular town or city, and if really you hit it off together, your new lover may very well ask you to pull up stakes and move. Think about this very seriously: Does your home mean more to you than a new lover? Would you really be prepared to pack up all of

your belongings and sell your home and relocate
to a new city? If the answer is no—or if you're
at all dubious—then don't answer personals from
Alaska if you live in Alabama, and vice versa.
Make up your mind whether you would be prepared to relocate for the sake of love or not, and,
if so, how far, and to what kind of city? If you're
a Bostonian, for example, could you really be
happy in Omaha?

Try to be realistic when you're defining what
kind of lover you want. Not all the wealthy men
in the world have dazzling looks, and not all of
the handsomest men have money. And ask yourself: Which is more important to me—security,
companionship, intellectual stimulus, shared interests, wealth, or sex? (And you don't have to be
embarrassed if you've answered "sex.")

2. *Don't rush your responses.* Don't hurriedly scour
   the papers on a lonely Saturday night, looking for
   an instant Mr. Right, or even an instant Mr. 75
   Percent Okay. Read them at your leisure, when
   you have plenty of time, listing the most likely
   ads logically and carefully, as if you were thinking
   of buying an automobile or an air-conditioning
   unit. Then make your choices based on your experience and your real needs. Be calm and busi-
   nesslike and totally honest with yourself. It's the
   only way that you'll discover the kind of lover you
   really want.

3. *Respond to more than one ad.* Many personals
   advertisers are very slow in responding, so sometimes it's sensible advice to answer two or three
   or even more.

4. *Take his ad with a grain of salt.* He will have
   worked very hard to promote his good bits and
   minimize his less attractive characteristics. Some
   of his problems he will omit from his ad alto-

gether (such as dandruff, or bad breath, or a shirt pocket crammed with nerd clips). But other problems he may well hint at, in case you're put off when you go out on your first date. Watch out for anything that suggests physical abnormality, or unusual sexual tastes. Also beware of the soulful and the self-obsessed, who can cause you long-lasting difficulties. That "sensitive, insightful soul" may well turn out to be a jealous obsessive who never takes no for an answer, and who follows you around for months. Also, don't be taken in by Cinemascope references to horseback riding on the seashore, or driving down the Pacific coast with the wind in your hair. These are optional experiences which you may or may not get when you answer this man's ad. You should be interested in *him*, not the scenery through which he rides (or drives).

5. *Write yourself an all-purpose response letter.* It will take you forever to answer every ad personally, apart from exhausting far too much of your emotional energy. Keep a standard reply that you can either copy out by hand, or (better still) store it in a word processor and print it out whenever you need it, adding the personal touch by hand addressing the envelope and writing "Dear Chuck . . ." or whoever it is, in fountain pen.

6. *If the ad carries a voice-mail number, call it.* You can tell a whole lot more from a voice than you can from a magazine ad. Does he *sound* like the kind of guy you're looking for? Does he have the kind of accent that appeals to you? Joyce Maynard said, "I would hear a person on the other end of the line, and if he didn't have an Oklahoma accent, I barely listened." If you're interested in the voice-mail message, listen to it two or three times, just in case you begin to pick up

something about his voice or his innuendo of which you're not too sure.

7. *When you meet him for the first time, discover as much as you possibly can.* Ask him lots of questions and listen attentively when he answers. Lonely men will almost invariably have a great deal to say. Ask him about his work and his leisure pursuits. Also—very importantly—try to put him into a social context. How many friends does he have and what are they like? Does he see very much of his family? Then you can check out his everyday tastes, by asking him what was the last book he read, and what was the last concert or theatrical performance he attended. Resist the temptation to tell him your life story, or to cry on his shoulder about your ex-lover or ex-husband, or how rotten fate has been to you. Instead, try to give him a clear idea of the kind of woman you are, and what you expect out of an intimate relationship.

8. *Be safety conscious about meeting new men, but don't be overcautious.* Just as a faint heart never won fair lady, paranoia never won handsome lover. Life has its risks, and dating a new man is one of them, whether you've met him through personal ads or through mutual friends or at a formal reception at the White House. Of course you should take sensible, streetwise precautions, and any man worth his salt will understand why you are being so careful. To start with, don't reveal your home address or telephone number. Arrange to meet for the first time at a mutually convenient bar or restaurant. I read one safety suggestion for the really nervous—and that was to "ask a friend to come along and sit at a nearby table, or even introduce her." But, to me, that suggestion was far too defensive. It has the smell

of fear, and if you're *that* much afraid, you shouldn't go at all. All you have to do is use your feminine judgment, and make sure that you're not alone with your date until you trust him as much as any woman can trust any man. When you're out on a date, particularly in the early stages of your relationship, make sure that at least one friend or member of your family knows where you are, who you're with, and when you're expected back—and make sure you date knows that they know. It doesn't take much: Just excuse yourself in the middle of dinner and say, "I must call my brother . . . he's expecting me round at eleven, to do some babysitting."

9. *Don't say maybe when you mean yes; and don't say maybe when you mean no.* If you like the man you've met, tell him that you'll call him, or that you'll leave a message for him, and do so, promptly. There are few things more damaging to a man's ego than to feel that you're umming and aahing about him, or that you're hedging your bets. If you really don't like him, then tell him that you've enjoyed his company, but, in all honesty, you don't think you two would hit it off. If you can't bring yourself to be so blunt, ask for his phone number and tell him that you'll call him. If he says "You won't call, will you?" say "Wait and see." And leave.

10. *Try placing your own personal.* If you can't find a man who sounds like the kind of man you're looking for, place an ad of your own. You can either do this yourself, or through one of numerous agencies, such as Together or Great Expectations or Prestige Partners. The best agencies don't come cheap, but their success record is extremely high, and they can save you a great deal of trial and error and a great deal of heart-

ache, particularly if you're inexperienced in the skill of finding a lover on the open market.

When you're writing your own personal, don't waste all of your expensive words describing yourself. Set yourself a limit of only three words—such as "tall, brunette DWF." The more you describe yourself, the more you limit your chances of getting a response. Forget about "sparkling," "vivacious," "academic," "sensual." You may be all of those things, but every extra adjective will deter at least ten extra would-be lovers. Remember that the men who are looking for love in the personals are just as hurt and shy and lonely as you are.

Instead, work out what kind of man you want, and tell them what you're looking for. A big corporation that advertises for sales directors doesn't waste its space telling the world how wonderful the corporation is. It simply says something like "multinational pharmaceutical company seeks talented, innovative sales director, aged 33–40, must be able to take responsibility of own nationwide sales department."

The way to write a successful personal is not to write an ad about you, but about the man you want to meet. If he's out there, he'll recognize himself in what you've written, and respond.

So how do you set about writing the perfect personal? It's really easy. If you answer all of these fundamental questions, you will have written a personal that is almost guaranteed a quick and genuine response: (1) What age partner do you prefer? (2) Are you prepared to relocate for marriage? (3) Would you like to meet somebody with children? (4) What standard of education do you prefer in your partners? (5) Smoker or nonsmoker? (6) What areas of interest is it important for you to share with your partner (music, dancing, sports, etc.)? (7) Do you have any physical preferences (tall, trim, athletic)? (8) Is there any special quality you look for in a lover (poetic, forthright, spontaneous, passionate)?

Place your ad, and from then on, you're on your own.

Quite a valuable guide to have beside you is the display ad for Zelda Fischer's Boston-based agency Gentlepeople. Zelda describes herself as "consultant to the world's fussiest single people." Her ad asks would-be lovers to match up to these criteria: "You are considerate, generous, intelligent, fun, romantic, successful—You are monogamous by nature—You're good to your parents—You love kids—You value your friends—You have a good sense of humor—You care about animals—You don't smoke or use drugs—You drink only in moderation—You want to be happily and permanently married."

I think Zelda would be the first to admit that few of us can match up to all of those criteria. Even those who take the thorns out of lions' feet have occasionally been known to shout at their aged grandmothers, and even those who drink in moderation have been known to tie one on from time to time. But she is absolutely right to place "consideration" and "generosity" at the head of her list. Consideration and generosity are the two most important qualities in a sexual relationship, and in the next chapter we shall see how you can use your consideration and your generosity in order to make yourself sexually irresistible to *all* men, without fail.

Of course there are plenty of other ways to make contact with single men apart from placing a personal.

Almost every major city has its lunch or supper clubs, where singles can meet one-to-one for lunch or an after-work drink, or in organized groups for evening dinner or dancing.

I have talked to many women who have successfully found lovers and/or husbands through organized lunch parties, but on the whole the personal ad or the personal introduction service still seems to me to be the most effective way of getting in touch with a man who will really light your fire. It can work out to be quite expensive, particularly if you use an agency such as Gentlepeople or Great Expectations or Together, but your romantic needs will be circularized around a far greater number of potential lovers, and so your chances of finding a suitable partner are proportionately far greater.

There is absolutely nothing demeaning or defeatist about turning to personal ads or personal introduction services in your search for a lover. I have talked to dozens of single women who have made the decision to use personals, and not one of them was anything but charming, sexy and more-than-delightful company. Their difficulty in finding a lover stemmed simply from the fact that their career or their social position made it almost impossible for them to meet the kind of man they really wanted. And, as one pretty, dark-haired divorcee told me, "Why should I have to put up with a second-best lover just because I can't get out and about every night to hunt down a first-class one?"

Here's a classic example of a single woman who found a new and highly exciting sex life through a personal introduction service:

Tina, 22, a qualified physical fitness instructor from Cranford, New Jersey: "I was engaged to my high school sweetheart, a guy named Tim. I always assumed that as soon as we had both finished college, we would get married and settle down and that would be that.

Looking back on our relationship now, I knew Tim wasn't a particularly good lover, although I didn't really know that when I was younger, because I'd never had any other man to compare. He would make love to me no more than once or twice a week, and usually after he'd had a few beers, which didn't make it very pleasant. He just used to climb on top of me, push himself in, and come, and that would be the end of it.

"One evening Tim was out of town on a job and a friend of mine invited me to a party. I went along, and it was a pretty swinging affair. I had a couple of glasses of champagne and really started to let my hair down. I danced with this tall, good-looking guy, and it didn't take him long to make it pretty obvious that he liked me a lot. His name was Mark, or Marcus. We danced real close to the slow numbers, and I realized that he had a hard-on, because he kept pressing it against my thigh.

"I was kind of startled at first, and didn't know what to do. But he kept on murmuring these compliments in my ear—telling me how beautiful I was, and how much he wanted to make love to me. After a while I accepted his hard-on as part of his flattery—it showed just how much I turned him on. I started to get real excited, and when he kissed me, I understood for the first time ever that I didn't have to marry Tim, there was no unwritten law that said that I had to. I understood for the first time ever that there are a whole lot of new and exciting men in the world.

"We couldn't use the bedrooms at the party because there were too many people around. Instead we found a den—well, more like a study, really, because it had a large leather-topped desk right in the middle of it.

"The trouble is, the floor was polished wood and there was no couch, only a highbacked leather armchair. But that didn't worry Mark at all. He kissed me, and he started to caress me through my dress. He was a great kisser. He didn't leave a single square inch of my tongue unsucked or a single tooth unlicked. And the way he kissed my neck and nuzzled my ears! He sent a shiver down my back that started at my neck and ended up right between my legs. He caressed my breasts until they felt as if they were tingling with electricity. I'd never felt anything like it.

"I remember saying something like 'We can't do it here . . . why don't you come back to my place?' But all he did was to. kiss me some more. Then he lifted me up so that I was sitting on the edge of the desk. There was a large old gilt-framed mirror on the wall next to the desk so that I could actually see myself looking over his shoulder. It felt kind of strange, and scary, too, but most of all it was exciting.

"He cleared the blotter off the desk, and he lay me back on that warm red leather, right on my back. He lifted my dress up over my hips, up to my waist. I was shivering with excitement . . . and I guess with fear, too! Underneath my dress I was wearing only pantyhose, no panties. He reached out with one finger and traced the outline of my cunt through the nylon gusset, and I could feel that I was very, very wet. He took his finger away and licked it, and it was then that I knew that this wasn't going to be the ordinary homestyle fucking that I was used to with Tim.

"He stripped off his necktie and his shirt. Then he unbuckled his belt and stepped out of his pants and his socks and his shorts. He climbed up onto the desk, and he was completely naked. He was quite heavily built but he was pretty fit, you could tell he worked out because his stomach was flat. He wasn't hairy, not like Tim. He was suntanned all over and very smooth, the color of caramel. He had black curly hair around his cock, but he'd obviously trimmed it, because it was short and very neat, not straggly. His cock was huge. It was fully hard, and I can remember how dark it was, almost purple, with a single shining drop of juice just oozing out of the hole at the end of it. I remember thinking that his balls swung like two pool balls in a red velvet bag.

"He leaned over me and kissed me. God, those kisses! He said I turned him on like no girl ever turned him on before. I laughed—although I was pleased that he'd said it. I said I didn't believe him. He took my hand and held it against his cock, and by now his cock was literally dripping juice onto the leather-topped desk. He said, 'That's all the proof you need.'

"I had never held a man's cock before, not like that. It felt so warm and silky-skinned, and yet hard and rubbery, too. I slid my hand up and down it, so that his juice smothered it from top to bottom. Then he took hold of my hand and guided it down between his legs, so that I could feel his hairy balls. 'Gently,' he warned me. Then he said, 'Do you know how good that feels? That feels good.'

"I loved the way he encouraged me to touch him like that. I even slid my finger between the cheeks of his bottom and stroked his anus. He shivered, and I knew that he liked that, too.

"Then he kissed me again, and lifted up my hips, and pulled down my pantyhose, right down to my knees, and then unrolled each leg, one at a time, until I was naked from the waist down. He raised my knees, and parted my thighs, and looked down at my cunt like he had discovered some fantastic treasure. He gently stroked all around it, touching and tickling at my clitoris. Then he opened up my lips with both hands, stretching me wide open. He slid his fingers into my actual cunt hole, and stretched that open, too. Tim had never done anything like that. Tim had never really *looked* at my cunt, let alone stretched it wide open.

"Mark said, 'Do you know what I see? I see hair like silk and pink wet flesh the color of coral and a dark secret place that leads somewhere mysterious.' I know what you're thinking. You're probably thinking, 'What bullshit.' But it didn't *sound* like bullshit and the way he said it sounded sincere, and at least he said something sexy and romantic, which was more than Tim ever did. Tim hardly ever said anything.

"He reached across the desk and picked up a condom. I watched him while he bit open the foil, and then fitted the condom over the head of his cock, and unrolled the shiny rubber all the way down his shaft. I helped him to tug it right down into his pubic hair, and at the same time I took hold of his balls, too, and rolled them gently in my right hand, and felt them tighten and lift.

"With my right hand, I took hold of his cock and guided it between my legs, until its big rubbery head was nestling between the open lips of my cunt. I lifted my head, and I could actually see myself in the mirror across the room, lying on the desk with my thighs wide apart, and my fingers curled around Mark's cock. I watched as his cock sank into my cunt, the whole way in. I was amazed how big his cock was, yet my cunt could take him all the way. It was fantastic to be able to watch what was happening as he fucked me. I couldn't just feel it, I could see it, too. I saw his balls swinging against the cheeks of my bottom. I saw my own fingers caressing them. I saw my own fingers clutching the hard suntanned cheeks of his ass.

"All the time, my bare bottom was making kissing noises on the leather-topped desk, and my cunt was so wet that it sounded as if I was playing in the tub.

"Mark thrust harder and harder. His muscles were shining with sweat and his cock felt gigantic. He said, 'I'm coming,' and I knew that I was almost coming, too. But for some reason I said, 'I want to see, I want to *see*.' I reached down and took his cock out of my cunt, and gripped it in both hands. I was so excited I kept feeling ripples all the way through my cunt. I was right on the very edge of coming. I rubbed Mark's cock up and down, up and down, as hard and as fast as I could, until suddenly he said 'Baby,' that was all he said. His cock throbbed, and the teat on the end of his condom suddenly popped up, filled with bubbly white sperm. His cock throbbed again, and I could see the sperm filling the whole head of his condom, like warm cream.

"I didn't come in the way that I'd always come before. It was more like a wave than anything else, a beautiful wave. My cunt was pressed against the leather top of the desk and I had made a sticky wet imprint on it. Mark kept on kissing me, and saying I was out of this world. I *felt* out of this world. I took hold of his cock and slid off his condom, and rubbed his cock up and down. It was all wet and rubbery and spermy, and I loved it. I suddenly understood that two people could do *anything* when they make love, so long as they both enjoy it. There don't have to be any inhibitions.

"As it turned out, I never saw Mark again. I found out about two days later that he was married, and I didn't want to date a married man. But he taught me so much about sex.

"After that, my relationship with Tim really began to fall apart, and we broke off our engagement. I didn't have a partner for over a year and a half. Every time I met a man, he always seemed so dull, so lacking in spontaneity, so lacking in passion. I kept thinking of Mark, fucking me on that leather-topped desk, his cock thrusting in and out of me. I kept thinking how much he had made me an equal partner in our lovemaking, too. All the men I met seemed to want to jump on me, or else they expected *me* to make all the running . . . nothing in between those two extremes. Then one evening I was talking to one of my friends, complaining that I couldn't find the kind of man I wanted, and she suggested joining a personal introduction agency. At first I thought she was joking, but she said that her own mother had found a fantastic new man through Together or one of those agencies, and that she'd never been so happy.

"So that's what I did. I registered with Together and another agency. They asked me what kind of partner I wanted and I was able to tell them. I wanted a man who was outgoing and spontaneous and passionate. I wanted a man who had very liberal views about women. Of course I had other requirements, like he had to be six-one or over, and reasonably interested in sports and aerobics, and I didn't want him older than 30.

"It took longer than I expected, and I went out on three totally terrible dates and two not-bad-but-not-terrific dates before I finally met Russell. He's a junior partner in a law firm, and he spends most of his days behind a desk, but he's just as keen on sports as I am . . . and he's *so-o-o* good looking. Well, I think he is! The main thing is, he's so good in bed. He's relaxed, and he's fun, and he never rushes me. And he likes it when *I* do things to him, too."

If you've never considered a personal ad or a dating agency, ask yourself the following questions.

1. Am I tired of being approached by men I don't like and always having to say "no" to them, when the kind of men I *do* like never, ever ask me out?
2. Am I tired of meeting good-looking men who immediately think they have the right to go to bed with me—and then, when I refuse, never call me again?
3. Am I tired of having relationships with men that never seem to go anyplace but downward?

4. Am I tired of going out with men I don't particularly like simply for the sake of companionship?

5. Am I tired of meeting men who seem to be everything I'm looking for, only to discover after a few months that they're not the people I originally thought they were?

6. Am I tired of looking for places where I can meet the same kind of people as me?

7. Am I tired of joining societies and sports clubs in the hope of meeting Mr. Right, only to end up feeling that I've wasted both time and money?

8. Am I tired of falling in love with men, only to discover that they're already married, or that I'm definitely not the only woman in his life?

9. At end of the day, have I been too busy at work to spend time looking for that special man?

10. Do I dislike the singles bar scene?

11. Do I feel that it's not particularly safe to go looking for a man at a club or a bar?

12. Am I tired of always being the spare wheel at dinners and parties and social get-togethers?

If your answer to any of these 12 questions is "yes," then you might seriously consider playing the personals or joining an introduction agency. If you do, and if you find that terrific lover you've always wanted, then please write and let me know about your romantic success!

NINE

How to Be Sexually Irresistible to Men

Tina, the young phys-ed instructor in our last chapter, discovered for herself the single most effective technique for making herself sexually irresistible to men. Because didn't she say: *"He likes it when I do things to him, too."*

Traditionally, men are supposed to be "in charge" when it comes to sex. Men are expected to be the seducers, and women are expected to be the seduced. Men, after all, are physically stronger than women. The act of sexual intercourse involves the man penetrating the woman's body. And whatever feminists say, much of the excitement that women derive from sex comes from being "taken" or "surrendering." It's a natural part of human psychology, and there is nothing that anybody can do about it except enjoy it.

Almost all of the blockbuster novels for women include scenes of rape, or—at the very least—scenes of forcible seduction. Not *real* rape, because real rape is horrendous, but fantasy rape, in which the rapist is invariably handsome. He may have designer stubble and designer sweat, but of course the reader doesn't have to sit in the shower for hours afterward, trying to wash off his smell.

In real life, however, men can be very reticent when it comes to sex. Although they are supposed to know everything about lovemaking and sexual technique and how to turn a woman on, not very many of them do. This has the effect either of making them overforceful when it comes to having sex, pushing their way into you with scarcely any foreplay and generally behaving like Visigoths on their evening off; or of making them so timorous in their sexual approaches that they never make you feel feminine and womanly, and fail to arouse you to the peaks of excitement that you expected and had every right to expect.

The way to make yourself sexually irresistible to the man you like is to play a very positive part in your lovemaking, while at the same time making him believe that he is the one who is sexually in charge. This technique has the doubly beneficial effect (a) of giving him extra excitement and fulfillment; and (b) of giving you extra excitement and fulfillment.

"If I had waited for Jimmy to give me oral sex, I think I would have had to wait until the next ice age," said Donna, a 27-year-old croupier from Reno, Nevada. "He was such a handsome guy, and he was real good in bed, except that he always did the same thing. He got on top of me and screwed me, and said, 'Oh babe, oh babe,' and that was all. I think he once put his finger up my snatch while we were sitting in the tub together, and he was so cautious and apologetic about it that I was amazed. Yet looking at him talking to the guys and flirting with all the girls, you would have thought he was the most sophisticated lover ever."

Assuming that the last few chapters have enabled you to find the man of your dreams, here are some of the techniques you can use to hold his sexual attention now and—if not forever—for a very long time to come.

Visual sex

Men can be sexually aroused very quickly by visual stimuli, much more quickly and much more strongly than women. Hence the enormous popularity of men's magazines crammed with nude girls and the comparative lack of success of women's magazines crammed with nude men (many of which are bought by homosexual men, in any case). A man can be erotically aroused simply by the sight of a woman's bottom or a woman's breast or a woman's vulva. I showed a photograph to 100 different men of a woman's vagina with her own red-varnished finger inserted into it. That was all—you couldn't see the women's face or the rest of her body or even determine her age. Of those 100 men, 86 percent thought that the photograph was "very erotic." I showed a photograph of a man's erect penis, clasped in his own muscular hand, to the female partners of the same 100 men. Their verdict: 23 percent thought it was "quite sexy," 55 percent said it had no sexual effect on them at all, and the remaining 22 percent said that it was a "turnoff."

Women take advantage of the way that men respond to visual stimuli every day of the week—with short skirts, figure-hugging tops, tight leggings, low décolletages, high-cut swimsuits. Perhaps the most famous use of visual stimuli was Sharon Stone's quick flaunting of her pantielessness in the movie *Basic Instinct*. I'm not suggesting for a moment that you walk around with no panties, opening your legs to every sexy man you meet, but you can use this and other visual teasers to keep your *own* man's sexual interest at a very high pitch.

The "no-panties" trick is one of the best. Actually, you don't even have to show your beau that you're not wearing any panties. All you have to do is whisper to him, halfway through the evening, "I forgot to put on my panties." Then see what effect it has on him. Nobody else will be able to see whether you're wearing any panties or not, but your man will stick to you like Crazy Glue for the rest of the evening—*just in case*—and believe me, he won't be able to think about anything else.

By the time you get home, you should have worked him up into a very attentive lather.

One sure-fire test of the effectiveness of the "no-panties" trick was a notorious British magazine advertisement in the 1960s showing a well-bred fur-clad woman in the back of a Rolls-Royce, immaculately dressed, with the caption: "Cynthia Isn't Wearing Panties." It caused a huge scandal and sold a great many pairs of pantyhose (which was what the small print in the advertisement eventually explained that Cynthia was wearing).

If you can devise a situation where you can show your man in public that you aren't wearing any panties, then by all means try it. Usually, it has a riveting effect! Here's my favorite account, from Kathy, 26, a blonde divorcee from Minneapolis. "I had met Jim through a personal dating service. We had dated six or seven times, and on the third date Jim had spent the night at my apartment, and we had slept together. To tell you the truth, it wasn't very good. I was scared of committing myself, I guess; and at the same time I was scared of losing him. I was floppy, I was awkward, our physical rhythms didn't seem to coincide at all, and I just couldn't get aroused. Jim must have felt like he was trying to make love to Raggedy Ann.

"Jim was polite. He isn't the kind of guy who would drop a woman just because she acted jittery in bed. We made love two or three times more, but *now* I was worried that he might be losing interest in me, and so I tried to make love with real passion and real aggression . . . you know, I tried to be *positive*. The trouble was, I was too aggressive, I wasn't acting naturally, and Jim just didn't seem to be able to handle that. Then my mother, of all people, said, 'Flirt with him. Show him that he turns you on, but leave the rest of it up to him. Men need to have their hands held.'

"Well, how right she was! The next time we met, a whole group of us concert lovers were having our picture taken in the Crystal Court in the IDS Building. Jim and I hadn't had a good day at all. That afternoon, I'd tried to tease him into bed, but he didn't seem to be interested. In fact, he said, 'What? So that you can rape me?' He sounded like he was joking, but only half-joking. I had the feeling that he was going to tell me over dinner that he didn't want to see me again.

"There were 70 or 80 of us in the Crystal Court, and while we were waiting for the photographer to set up his cameras I had an idea. Pretty desperate idea, I have to admit! I excused myself for a few minutes and went to the ladies' restroom. I took off my panties and put them into my purse. Then I went back and joined the group.

"We were all pretty much squashed tight together. Jim was standing right behind me, with his hands on my shoulders. I leaned back and whispered over my shoulder, 'I brought you a souvenir.' He said, 'A souvenir. What of?' And I said, 'Today . . . this photograph.' He said, 'What is it?' And I said. 'My panties. They're in my purse.' And I opened up my purse so that he could see them.

"He stared at me for a long time. Then he said, 'You took them off!' But he was smiling and I could tell that he was imagining me naked underneath my skirt, and I could tell that I had hooked his interest. And all I said was, 'Did I?'

"When the time came for the photograph, I felt Jim pressing up very close behind me. People were smiling and nodding at us, and we were smiling back, too.

Especially when Jim lifted my skirt at the back, and slid his hand in, between my legs. He felt my bare bottom and *I* felt his cock rising up. Right there, right in the middle of Crystal Court, among all of those people.

"He opened the lips of my pussy with his finger, and slid it up inside me. Right up, as far as he could go. And all the time they were taking that picture, I was having my pussy massaged by Jim's finger. That's why we both have this real strange expression on our face, like we've been smoking wacky tobaccy or something."

For Kathy, that incident in the IDS Building in Minneapolis was only the beginning of something very exciting—what she called "a program of continuing excitation." She took the opportunity again and again to give Jim sexually tantalizing treats—like cleaning his apartment on Saturday mornings wearing nothing but a man-sized checkered shirt and bending over, of course, to plug in the Hoover, so that he accidentally on-purpose glimpsed her bare bottom. Like accidentally-on-purpose allowing him to see her while she was sitting on the toilet. Like asking him to shave her armpits for her. She used a whole variety of little things that made him think that he was in control, that he was being masterful and protective and "in-charge," while she was small and vulnerable and feminine.

Many women don't realize that a man can be attracted to them by the simple act of being asked to fasten the top back button on their dress, or by opening the overtightened lid of a jar of pickles. You think I'm joking? The first gives them an opportunity to demonstrate their sensitivity and their caring; the second gives them an opportunity to demonstrate their strength. If I were you, I'd tighten up every jar of pickles you own, just to give the man in your life the joy of opening them for you. Men don't often have the chance to prove themselves in battle any more. A jar of pickles makes a small but happy substitute.

Another way of giving the man in your life some visual excitement is to wear sexy underwear. These days, the kind of underwear that was once thought only suitable for hookers or Las Vegas strippers is available in most chain stores, or by mail order from several reputable companies. Most men are aroused by the sight of a woman in black stockings and garter belt (with or without panties), and you can buy a stunning variety of panties, from lacy G-strings to silky French step-ins to split-crotch panties that offer some extremely flirtatious glimpses whenever you walk (and particularly when you bend over).

Some women have reported great success with "bondage wear," such as black leather corsettes that leave your nipples exposed, or black leather bikinis that support your bare breasts with nothing but studded straps. The most erotic item (judging from the response that it received from those men whose lovers were daring enough to wear it) was a leather domina thong—a buckle-up G-string which was split open at the crotch to reveal the wearer's vulva, and fitted with a tight metal chain that ran from front to back, between the labia.

Other items of erotic clothing that aroused a high level of visual response were rubber miniskirts and rubber panties, and a seemingly demure black rubber corsette which covered the breasts and the vulva, but that revealed (when the wearer turned around) a completely bare bottom.

Many of the women with whom I discussed the techniques of visually arousing their men were shy about showing themselves off. "He'll think I'm a whore" was one anxiety. Another was: "I don't like my figure very much. I don't want to show it off."

The answer to the first objection is that with very

few exceptions men *don't* think that their women are whores if they treat them to visual stimulation. Quite the opposite. Your man will be delighted by what you are doing, especially if you make it plain that you have never exposed yourself like this with any other man (even if this isn't strictly true) and that what you are showing him is for his eyes only.

Obviously you know your man better than I do, and you will be able to judge for yourself what his reaction is going to be. But most men would adore it if their women were more daring in what they wore, and more flirtatious in the way that they wore it.

As far as being embarrassed about your figure is concerned, the only answer to *that* is: Don't be. Your lover is attracted to you because of who you are and what you look like. If you dress sexy and act sexy, and make the very best of what you've got (or haven't got) then you don't have anything to worry about. You're you. The very fact that you're reading this book is proof that you're sexy and interested in finding out how to show your lover that you want to arouse him.

Even the Top Ten sexiest women of all time had very much less than perfect figures. I'm always being told by anxious women: "I wish I had a figure like Marilyn Monroe/Jayne Mansfield/Sharon Stone/Demi Moore." But the plain truth is that none of those women could be described as physically perfect—far from it. Marilyn Monroe had a deep chest but quite small breasts. It was only because she wore good bras and cleavage-flattering dresses that she gave the lasting (but quite mythical) impression that she was busty. If you're small breasted, you can do the same. Jayne Mansfield was large breasted but also very heavy hipped and (in her later days) quite fat, too. That didn't turn off her husbands and lovers. It was the sexiness and the warmth of personality that she exuded that made her attractive.

Here's a very telling excerpt from a conversation I had with 41-year-old Darryl, an architect from Oxnard, California, about the erotic effect that his new girlfriend Susan had on him. Susan was a 36-year-old divorcee from Pasadena whom Darryl had met through a personal introduction service. (A few weeks after this conversation, she became his wife.)

"I went through to the kitchen to make early-morning coffee for both of us. It was a beautiful morning. The sun was shining, the patio doors were open, the net curtains were blowing in the breeze. I came back into the bedroom, and Susan was sitting up in bed, reading the Sunday paper. Her hair was all tangled, she wasn't wearing makeup. She was wearing nothing but a pale yellow pajama top. The pajama top had ridden up on her hips, and the sheet had been dragged down, so that her sex was exposed. Her thighs were slightly parted, and so the lips of her sex had parted too. She has nothing more than a little blonde tuft of hair just above her sex . . . she keeps the rest of it hairless because of swimsuits. I stood in the doorway looking at her, and she was so damned pretty, and so relaxed, and yet there she was, showing me her bare sex, showing me her clitoris and right inside herself, where she was all pink like sugar candy, and I can tell you here and now that I loved her then more than I'd ever loved her before, and knew that she wasn't ashamed to expose herself in front of me. I had a boner that put the CNN Tower to shame, and I climbed onto that bed and I dipped my head down, and I gave her a kiss and a lick on her sex, and that wasn't just the start of another lovemaking session—that was the start of a whole relationship."

Hair or bare? The attraction of depilation

Out of all of the sexual techniques that I have discussed over the past decade, pubic shaving (or waxing, or electrolysis, or other depilation) has attracted some of the greatest interest (and appreciation). Although I am quite aware that there is a body of feminist opinion that holds that women shouldn't shave off their pubic hair simply to satisfy the unnatural lusts of their menfolk, the fact remains that those women who have tried it now and again as a means of rekindling sexual interest in their lovers have found it to be stunningly effective. In a long-term sexual relationship, or a long-term marriage, shaving off your pubic hair will suddenly make your lover look at you with new eyes—after all, a little frisson of freshness never did anybody's sex life any harm.

If you don't happen to like it (or if *he* doesn't particularly care for it) then you can always grow it back again within a matter of two to three weeks. And if you do like it, you can either grow it back and then shave it again two or three months later, or keep on shaving it. If you prefer to keep your vulva permanently bare, of course, you will have to have treatment by electrolysis to destroy the hair roots.

"Ever since you suggested it in one of your books, I've used a depilatory cream on my pubic area as a matter of course," wrote Gina, a 32-year-old divorcee from Phoenix. "I like it because it feels clean and free, and all of my boyfriends like it. I'd go further than that, and say that they go ape about it. I've had four sexual relationships since I was divorced. Three of the men I met through my personal introduction service and one by chance in the bar of the Biltmore. All four relationships have been exciting and different, and they've done wonders to restore my self-confidence. I'm not a slender woman, by any means. I'm very heavy breasted. But all of those four men said that I was by far the sexiest woman they had ever met in their lives. And to think that my ex-husband called me frigid!"

Some women are reticent about shaving because they feel that it will make them look childlike, and that there is something perverted about a man who is aroused by the sight of girlish genitalia. Although it would be wrong to ignore the fact that there are people who have a sexual interest in children, the sexual stimulus that a man derives from the bare-shaved vulva of a mature woman is quite different.

There are two main reasons why pubic shaving arouses men so much. The first is that it offers them a completely unobscured look at their lover's vulva. They can see your lips and your clitoris without any difficulty whatsoever. The second is that you have done that crucial thing in making yourself irresistible—you have taken a positive step to expose yourself sexually to him, to show him that you want him to see your vulva (and, by implication, to touch it, too). You have given him the very stimulating feeling that you have surrendered yourself to him, whereas in reality it is you who have taken the first step. A woman who shaves off her pubic hair for a man is giving him the clearest and strongest signal possible that she is sexually attracted to him and that she wants him. The razor speaks for itself. No words are necessary.

There are other benefits to shaving yourself, too. Women who have removed their pubic hair report a quantum increase in the number of times that their lovers have given them oral sex, or *cunnilingus*.

Rachael, 28, a jeweler from San Antonio, Texas, said, "I trimmed my pubic hair right from my high-school days because of my high-cut swimming suits. But one day I read in your book that men find it real attractive if you take it all off, so I thought, what the hell, and I did. It was just as easy as trimming the edges, after all. I liked it myself, I still do, I think it's neater and cleaner and I wouldn't go back to having pubic hair, not again. After all, women shave their armpits and nobody thinks it's weird, do they?

"When I went to bed that night, I showered and toweled myself and came into the bedroom. My boyfriend Stan was sitting up in bed finishing off a project for work. He looked up and he did a classic double-take. That project was dropped on the floor quicker than you could say "Gillette!" He said, 'You shaved your pussy. That's fantastic.' He reached out for me, and pulled me down onto the bed. He couldn't stop kissing me and touching and stroking my pussy. He said, 'I love it, I love it. I have to kiss it.'

"He opened my legs wide and he kissed and licked and sucked my pussy all over . . . not just inside, but everywhere. He sucked my whole lips right into his mouth, and licked all around every which where. He buried his whole face in me, as if he hadn't eaten in a week, and he couldn't get enough of me. His tongue started flicking at my clitoris, and all the time he kept up this gentle tugging, sucking pressure too, trying to take as much of my pussy into his mouth as he could.

"I had one of the fastest orgasms ever, and it was amazing. The whole world went dark, I swear it, and afterward I went on twitching and jumping for what seemed like *hours*. Stan lifted his head and his whole face was smothered in juice. He said, 'You're amazing. I could have you for breakfast, lunch, and dinner.' I reached with my hand into the fly of his pajama pants, and found that they were full of sperm. He'd climaxed at the same time as me, without even being touched."

Some women are reluctant for their lovers to give them oral sex. They feel that it's vaguely "dirty" or "not very nice," and they can't imagine how a man could enjoy licking and kissing their vagina, especially when it's all wet and juicy. In fact, most men are highly aroused by giving cunnilingus—by the smell, by the taste, by the wetness, and by the way in which it allows them very accurately to sense how close their women are to orgasm. There can't be any more sensitive way of judging how stiff a woman's clitoris is than by running the tip of your tongue up and down it.

I have often recommended to men who are suffering from temporary impotence that they should indulge for a while in much more oral sex. Not only is it arousing in itself, but it means that he can bring his lover to orgasm whether he has managed to achieve an erection or not.

If you have any reservation about oral sex, do try to overcome them. In fact, try to encourage your man to give you oral sex, both by shaving your pubic hair and by putting yourself in a position where he can hardly refuse.

"My husband loves it when I climb astride his chest when he's lying in bed, and open up my cunt with my fingers. He always says he's tired or he doesn't feel like it, but I've never known him to resist taking a quick lick . . . and after he's taken one quick lick, he has to finish the whole meal!"

I have had a few letters from women whose pubic hair is quite thick and who have difficulty in keeping their vulva completely bare. The answer for them is simply to keep their pubic hair thinned out with thinning scissors and very closely trimmed—not so short that it's stubbly, but short and sparse enough not to conceal their vulva from the loving gaze of their loving men.

Oral sex

There is no question about it, men love having their cocks sucked. It feels delightful and unlike sexual intercourse they can actually watch it happening (visual

stimulus yet again). The most common single com-
plaint that I receive from men about their sex lives is
that their wives or girlfriends won't give them oral
sex—or, if they *can* be persuaded to, do it with obvious
distaste, and not very often.

I cannot emphasize enough that if you want to be
irresistible to the man you love, you must think seriously about giving him frequent and skilful oral sex. I
met a feminist author who said that women shouldn't
give oral sex to men because it meant having to kneel
to them. Physically speaking, it hardly ever means that
at all, because oral sex is mostly performed in a lying-
down position, with the woman on top. But it doesn't
mean that psychologically or morally, either. When a
woman is giving a man oral sex, she is in total control
of his sexual arousal, of how stimulated he feels, of
when he is going to reach his climax (if at all), and of
what is going to happen when he ejaculates.

You may think now that taking your lover's cock into
your mouth is a servile gesture, but after you've become a little more experienced at it, you'll quickly grow
to realize that it's one of the best ways for you to assert
yourself sexually and to control the pace and the intensity of your sex life.

If you don't particularly feel like intercourse but he
does, you can give him oral sex until he climaxes, and
then he won't feel cheated. If you're usually slow to
become sexually aroused, you can give him slow oral
sex, keeping your stimulation to a minimum, while you
either masturbate yourself with your other hand, or
(better still) sit on top of him in the 69 position, and
encourage him to lick your cunt while you suck his
cock. You can judge how hard to stimulate him by the
degree of stimulation that he is giving you. Then, when
you're ready, you can turn around and sit on top of his
cock and again control the stimulus he's giving you by
adjusting the speed and rhythm of your fucking, and

by leaning forward (less stimulation) or sitting upright (more stimulation).

Despite the fact that *you* have been at the reins of the whole sexual act from beginning to end, your lover will never feel that he has been anything but manly and "in charge." He will feel proud, sexually confident, and he will be more than looking forward to the next time, believe me.

Some women are worried that they don't know how to give a man oral sex and that they might somehow do it wrong, and wind up frustrating him more than arousing him. Really—there's nothing to it, provided that you remember that the slang terms "blow-job" and "cocksucking" are both inaccurate. You should never blow into a man's penis, just as he should never blow into your vagina. There is a small but real risk that you could introduce an air embolism into the bloodstream, with fatal consequences. You can suck your man's cock, by all means, but not too hard, which will cause him nothing but irritation or even pain.

Take his penis in your hand, and simply put your mouth around the head. If it's already hard, roll down his foreskin (if he has one) and run your tongue around the corona or ridge, probing into the opening with your tongue tip and flicking the thin web of skin (the frenum or frenulum) just below it. You can gently and rhythmically suck and at the same time swirl your tongue around and around. Then you can suck it so that it slides out from between your lips, ending each suck with a kiss.

How far you can take his cock into your mouth depends on how far you *want* to take it into your mouth, and what position you're in. Even today, I'm still asked about "deep throating" and how it's done. Although Linda Lovelace was later to decry the circumstances in which she made the movie *Deep Throat,* the fact remains that the oral sex technique she popularized is still famous (or notorious, depending on your point of view).

"Deep throating" is the act of taking the entire length of your man's erect penis into your mouth, right up to the balls, so that the head of his penis will actually slide into your throat. The main difficulties to overcome are the urge to gag whenever any object enters your throat, and breathing. A sword swallower can breathe around the blade of a sword, but a woman can't breathe around a fat, erect cock.

Linda Lovelace overcame the gagging by practice— putting her finger down her throat and then training herself not to swallow when an object was inside her throat.

"Then I realized the only way full penetration could be achieved was to position myself so my mouth and throat were in a straight line. I managed this best by positioning myself on my back, lying on the bed with my head hanging over the edge of the mattress. The man kneels on the floor facing me and sticks his prick into my mouth. It slides easily into my throat in this position, and he can fuck away.

"I kept taking it deeper and deeper, establishing rhythm with the strokes of the cock. On his back stroke, I'd take a breath. From here, it was a matter of accommodating size, but once the cock passes the throat muscles, length is no problem."

Linda Lovelace recommended "deep throating" for women who don't much care for the taste of semen. "The only way you know he's coming is by the muscular spasms you feel in your mouth from his cock."

Of course, "deep throating" is not the kind of sexual technique that you'll feel like attempting until you know your lover really well, and you're quite secure in your relationship. It takes practice, concentration and a great deal of mutual trust. I know hardly any women who have tried it, and even fewer who have enjoyed it.

Personally I think it belongs in the movie archives rather than the bedroom.

You don't necessarily have to fellate your lover until he climaxes. Licking and sucking his cock is a good straightforward way to revive a flagging erection, or to get him hard in the first place.

Yolande, 33, a history teacher from Cincinnati, said: "There is no feeling that gives me more satisfaction than taking my lover's soft cock into my mouth, and then gradually feeling it stiffen and well, until it's almost bursting."

You should concentrate most of your stimulation on the head of the cock, where most of his erotic nerve endings are located, but he will enjoy you sliding your tongue down the shaft, and even sucking the shaft, and licking and sucking at his balls. Between his balls and his anus is a very sensitive area called the perineum, and a little bit of oral attention to that will give him a disproportionate amount of pleasure.

To stimulate him toward a climax, you may need to rub his cock with your hand as well as lick and suck him with your mouth. Keep up a rhythmical rubbing, gentle but strong. Don't keep stopping and starting, or changing your grip, or altering rhythms. Think how you like your clitoris to be stimulated—consistently and *per*sistently. Sexual climaxes are built up slowly and gradually, without constant distraction. And don't give up if he seems to be taking a long time to climax. Just keep at it and enjoy it. I have talked to women who take anything up to 20 minutes to be manually stimulated to orgasm, while others can climax within four or five, or even less.

Although men adore oral sex, you may have to do it together three or four times before you get to know each other's rhythms and responses. Eventually, you will feel his balls tighten and his whole cock swell to maximum hardness. You will also be able to feel telltale upward movements of his pelvis, which will indicate that he is very close to ejaculating.

How you deal with that ejaculation when it happens is entirely up to you. A lot of women enjoy swallowing it. After all, it's only a slightly gelatinous mixture of proteins and simple sugars, with a slightly salt/sweet/bleachlike taste. If you don't feel like swallowing it, however, you can exploit its visual stimulus for all you're worth, by directing it on to your face and hair, or smearing it all over your breasts and nipples. He won't forget *that* in a hurry.

Oral sex is such an important part of making yourself irresistible to the man you love that you ought to make a point of thinking about doing it at least twice a week—and not just at bedtime, either. What about those times when he's just come out of the shower, and he's sitting around in his bathrobe, watching TV? What about the middle of the night, when he's asleep? What about waking him, by sucking his cock? What about surprising him in the tub and giving him a licking? In terms of the sexual appreciation and affection that your spontaneous acts of oral sex will earn you from the man you love, you will be making one of the best investments of your life. And that's a promise.

Any caveats? Well, yes, to be realistic. Watch out for the man who forces you to go down on him when you really don't want to, or the man who holds your head when he's climaxing, so that you don't have any choice but to swallow his sperm. Tell any man who tries to do either of those things to you that oral sex is an act of love, not an act of subservience. Show him this book, if you have to. And if he ever tries to do it again, show him the door. There is always room in every sexual relationship for a certain amount of teasing and roughness and coercion and biting and playacting. There is never any room for one person forcing their own preferences onto another against their will.

There are many variations to straightforward cocksucking. One of the most startling is to fill your mouth full of crushed ice before you go down on your lover. Another is to rub his cock with mint-flavored toothpaste, which will give him an interesting stinging sensation as you suck him and masturbate him.

It may sound less than sophisticated, but one of the very best of oral sex techniques was described to me by Karen, a 17-year-old high school student from Schaumburg, Illinois: "I liked my boyfriend Paul a whole lot, but I wasn't ready for intercourse—partly because I didn't want to risk getting pregnant, and partly because I want to save myself for somebody I truly love. I guess that sounds pretty stupid—saving yourself for somebody you truly love, when you've been sucking other guys' cocks. But they expect it, you know? They expect a blow at the very least; or else they don't go out with you no more. It's like getting a blow is some kind of American fetish, you know?

"Anyhow, I went out with Paul and he was getting all hot and heavy and trying to get into my jeans, you know? I tried to put him off by saying I was hungry, but of course that was the worst thing I ever could have said to a guy like Paul. Before I could even *blink,* he had opened up his zipper and taken out his big stiff dick. 'Something for a girl with a healthy appetite,' he said.

"Don't get me wrong. I liked him, and he turned me on. I didn't mind giving him a blow. In fact, I *wanted* to give him a blow. There's no feeling on this whole planet like having a guy's big stiff dick in your mouth and thinking 'I could give this guy infinite pleasure or infinite pain.' Like—he thinks he's such a big macho lover, with his dick in your mouth, but all you have to do is bite him hard, and what's he going to do about that? Men are strong, for sure. But they're vulnerable, too. I think God knew what he was doing when he gave men such vulnerable pricks and balls.

"Anyway, I wanted to give Paul a blow, but I wanted to show that I didn't care *too* much. So I didn't bother to take the gum out of my mouth. It was blueberry-flavored Bubblicious. It has that kind of sharp berry flavor, right? It goes good with the taste of dick. I mean, originally, I did it out of contempt, right? But when I was actually sucking him, I found that he *liked* it, because I could loop the gum in a thin string around his dick, or stretch it wide and cover the whole of his dick head with it, or else I could force it up against the hole in his dick, or tie it around his balls. He loved it. He loved it so much. And I loved it, too, because he was *s-o-o-o* turned on.

"He came in my mouth, and I loved it. All over my tongue, thick warm sperm. And I chewed it into my gum, all mixed up together, so that for a while there I was chewing sperm-flavored Bubblicious—definitely a flavor they should try to market!"

Since Karen told me about her bubblegum technique, I have discovered several other women who enhance their oral sex with unusual additives. One recommended a mouthful of strawberry-creme chocolates; another swore by dry breadcrumbs ("They drive him crazy"). Yet another said that she always kept a mug of warm chocolate beside the bed when she gave her lover oral sex. One swallow made her mouth unusually hot, and her lover just adored plunging his penis into such a soft, wet, hot, sweet, chocolatey mouth. Other suggestions included raspberries ("You flick and tumble them around his prick with your tongue, and then squash them up against his prick hole") and shortbread ("He can't resist having grainy, half-chewed shortbread smoothed and rubbed all around his cock").

You will eventually discover the oral technique that pleases your lover the most. But never be afraid to experiment or to try surprises. And never be afraid to act spontaneously and take out his cock when he's least expecting it. The most successful sexual relationships always have an element of teasing and flirtation and surprise.

Some men are not used to spontaneous displays of sexual affection, and will give you a very negative, stuffy response when you try to open their fly. The only way to deal with *that* kind of reaction is to shrug it off, and kiss them, and say "Your loss," and give them one more affectionate squeeze of their cock. This will show (a) that you're not at all embarrassed about what you've done—and why should you be? (b) that you still feel just the same way toward them; and (c) that you're quite happy to do it again, once they've had the opportunity to go away and think about it (and probably kick themselves, too, for acting in such an inhibited way).

Even when there's no opportunity for oral sex, give your lover an occasional intimate fondle. In bed, maybe, when he's reading or watching television. Or in the car, when he's driving. Come up behind him when he's cooking or washing dishes or cleaning his car, and reach around and massage his cock through his pants. It only takes a moment, and he'll probably protest. But he won't ever forget it. It's all part of the same technique of taking positive steps to stir up your sex life, but steps your lover won't ever perceive as domineering.

When you fondle his cock through his pants, he'll think that you find him sexually irresistible. If you can convince him of that, then he'll think that *you* are irresistible, too. It's as simple as that.

Videos and photography

Today's cameras and camcorders are a boon for lovers who want to make a record of their own lovemaking and play it back to themselves as a stimulus for further sex.

Most men find it very erotic to take photographs and videos of the woman they love, and you will certainly make yourself irresistible if you suggest to your lover that he takes some erotic pictures and videos of you.

One strict word of warning, however: Ask yourself if you can be sure that you can trust him, before you allow him to take pictures of you. You won't want explicit photographs or videos circulated to other people after your relationship has ended. If you are in any doubt at all, don't try it. But if you do believe that you can trust him, then go ahead, wholeheartedly. You too can be a porno star!

Here's Alison, a 25-year-old legal research assistant from St Louis: "Steve was about my fifth date through a personal introduction service. We hit it off from the moment we met. He was a keen photographer—his apartment was filled with all of the pictures he'd taken, and some of them were so beautiful . . . his pictures of Defiance and Hannibal and Sainte Genevieve were absolutely haunting.

"We slept together on our third date. I think I was pretty much convinced by then that we were going to stay together for a very long time. When we wanted to talk, we talked like old friends. When we didn't want to talk, there was no uncomfortable silence, we just sat and enjoyed each other's presence. In other words, I was sure that even if we didn't get married our relationship was going to last as long as a marriage.

"One morning I suggested to Steve that he should take some pictures of me just the way he saw me. Some nudes, if he wanted. So that's what he did. I took off all of my clothes and he photographed me all around the house. I love this one . . . I'm lying on the bed naked, with my legs open, so that you can see my cunt and everything, completely bare, and I've got one hand just slightly tugging the lips of my cunt open . . . but with the other hand, I've wound all the sheets around my head like an Arab yashmak, so my face is hidden. It's a really sexy and mysterious photograph. In fact it's so good that Steve had it framed and we've hung it up on the bedroom wall. I'm not ashamed of looking sexy.

"He took lots of other pictures of me, and they're all real artistic and beautiful. He's such a good photographer. Look at this one, I'm wearing a crown of roses, and I'm holding my bare breasts up, and my whole cleavage is filled with roses. And this one, I'm lying on my back here, with my legs in the air, and the whole bed is strewn with 30 or 40 cucumbers . . . I forget how many Steve bought. But I'm pushing one of the cucumbers halfway up my cunt . . . and look at my face, I look absolutely ecstatic. You can't call this pornography, this is *art*. And look at this . . . Steve titled it 'Lunch.' I'm down on my hands and knees on the kitchen table, stark naked, with my bottom lifted, and I have this submarine sandwich sticking out of my asshole, it had lettuce and tomatoes, and salami in it, and everything. Steve had to fit a condom over it and smother it with KY to get it up my ass.

"He took so many pictures, and I took some, too. I took one of Steve's prick, surrounded in whipped cream, with a cherry on top. Taking pictures made us look at ourselves differently. I mean we really learned to *look* at each other, and think what it was that turned us on. My favorite picture of Steve is this one. You can only see his ass and his balls and half of his erect prick. He's holding open the cheeks of his ass with his fingers, and there's a beautiful daisy sticking out of his asshole. I call it 'The Flower Picture to End All Flower Pictures.'

"And this one, too: This was my first experiment with high-speed film. I sucked Steve's prick and then he masturbated himself, and I've caught his prick right at the instant of climax. Look at that, the sperm's just squirting out at the end of his prick. It's already made a kind of loop."

Because of Steve's professional expertise, Alison's photographs were exceptionally high quality. But when your date takes pictures of you, or you take pictures of him, they don't have to be exhibition standard. Polaroids are good because you don't have to send them away to be developed, although their sharpness and quality leaves something to be desired, and what everybody wants from a sex picture is sharpness and quality.

June is a 32-year-old caterer from Hartford, Connecticut—blonde and busty and very pretty. A divorcee ("I can't think why he left me—*I* wouldn't have left me"), she met a new partner through the personals, an insurance agent named Jeff. For the first three months, June and Jeff got along together "like a fire on fire." They made love, but June felt that Jeff was very sexually inhibited. He never attempted anything more than the most straightforward lovemaking, and he seemed to find it difficult to tell her how he felt about her. She wondered if he were afraid of being rebuffed, or ridiculed.

June began to worry that their sexual relationship "wasn't really going anyplace at all." Jeff seemed to have a block about sexual variations—even oral sex—although he continued to insist that he loved June dearly, and that he was looking forward to a long-term relationship.

She wrote to me and discussed the problem on the telephone. Then I talked to Jeff. To cut a long and sensitive story short, Jeff had been living alone for three years and had been relying for sexual relief entirely on masturbation, using pornographic magazines and videos as a stimulus. Although he had been involved in a very active sex life before his three years of isolation, he had now become used to pornography as his sole means of achieving sexual satisfaction. For that reason, it was difficult for him to develop a full and varied sex life with a living, breathing, opinionated, sexually hungry woman. It was a question of adjustment, more than anything else.

My suggestion was that June should prompt Jeff to take a sexy video of her. In this way, he would subconsciously be reminded that the pictures in pornographic magazines and videos are just erotic images, whereas June was not only an erotic image but a real-life woman. It would help him to make the change from *observation* to *participation*—quite apart from which, it would be lots of erotic fun for both of them.

Fun, incidentally, is the most important ingredient of sexual enjoyment. I have read scores of deeply serious sexual manuals and watched dozens of "sensitive and thoughtful" sex-instruction videos—and none of them have mentioned the simplest of facts, that fucking is fun. It's not just a way of "communicating on the highest level, physically and emotionally." It's extremely pleasurable, it's almost always harmless (provided you take the right precautions), and it's very, very stimulating. Time and time again, I have advised couples with sexual hang-ups to stop worrying about their climaxes and their technique and to concentrate instead on doing what they enjoy—on having fun.

June said: "Jeff took a video of me and at first I was very self-conscious and awkward. I kept waving at the camera and saying things like, 'This is me, taking off my bra.' But Jeff said nothing at all, just kept following me around with the camcorder, and in the end I started to relax. The video starts with me taking off my clothes in the dressing room. There are mirrors on the closet doors and so you can see three images of me. I like that sequence, I think it's really good. I take off my bra and step out of my panties, and then I turn around and around in front of the mirrors, naked. Then I press my face right up to one of the mirrors and kiss my reflection, and lick it, tongue-to-tongue. Then I press my breasts up to my reflection, nipples squashed against nipples.

"I stroke my body and act all sexy and dreamy. Then I sit down on the rug in front of the mirrors and start to caress my hair and my breasts. I open up my legs and start to rub my pussy. You can see three of me, rubbing my pussy. I slide my middle finger inside my pussy, sliding it in and out. Jeff did a fantastic close-up: my pussy fills the whole screen practically, and you can see my finger sliding in and out, all sticky and wet.

"Then I leave the dressing room and go to the bedroom. I lie on the bed and start squeezing my breasts and rubbing my pussy and moaning. I don't care for that sequence too much—it looks too much like one of those porno videos. I like the silent sequences, they're almost like a dream, and they're much more romantic. You can tell what Jeff really felt for me, because he keeps coming in with this fantastically close focus, it's like the whole camera wants to eat me up. He wanted to get to *know* me, you can feel it. He wanted the two of us to join together.

"I take two dildoes out of the nightstand drawer. They're big and veiny and pink and they look just like real cocks except they don't have a man attached. I used to use them before I met Jeff.

"There's a long close-up sequence of me kissing and licking this dildo; the close-up is *so* close that it looks like I'm kissing and licking a real cock. I close my eyes and open my mouth and take the dildo right into my mouth, and suck it. Then you see me with a dildo in each hand, massaging my breasts and nipples, around and around, until my nipples are real hard.

"At last you see my legs wide apart and my pussy open. I never saw my pussy before—not like that, anyway, and it was quite a shock. But then I watched my own fingers pulling my pussy open, and I saw my own clitoris, and my own pussy hole, brimming with juice, and I thought: that's beautiful, that's really beautiful, that's my womanhood, that's my sex, that's what I am.

"Then you see this huge pink dildo pushing into my pussy hole, and you can hardly believe that it's going to fit in, but it does. It slides in and out, and you can see the juice bubbling up all around it, and then you can see my fingers, pushing it right in, right the way up to the hilt.

"I lift up my legs a little more, so that you can see my asshole, and Jeff takes an incredible close-up, you can see my pussy-juice trickling down to my asshole, so that it's all red and shiny. Then the other dildo appears from the other side of the screen, and you can see me forcing it into my ass—you can see my ass opening up, and kind of wincing, and then the whole dildo slowly—slowly—pushing its way up, and my asshole stretched so wide that you can hardly believe it. Right up to the hilt, seven inches long and three inches wide.

"So I've got two dildoes up inside me, and I'm sliding both of them in and out, and the camcorder's right up close to them, so that you can see every single detail. And this goes on and on, quicker and quicker, and at last I clench my thighs together, and that's my orgasm, and there's a whole blurry sequence, where I'm shaking. Then you can see me squeezing the dildo out of my ass, and my asshole's still red and juicy and sore looking and gaping wide, but it's a *very* sexy moment. Then the other dildo comes out of my pussy, just as juicy. And that's the end.

"Well, it's the end of the video, but it isn't the end of what happened. Because after Jeff put down the camcorder, he stripped off his clothes, and he climbed onto the bed, and his cock was sticking out like a rocket. He was so turned on that he fucked me like crazy, like he'd never fucked me before. He fucked my pussy, and then took out his cock and he fucked my mouth, and then he turned me around on my stomach and he fucked my asshole. He was pulling my ass cheeks wide apart with both hands and he was shoving his cock up my ass until I thought I was going to scream, it felt so good. And his balls kept thumping against my pussy, I could feel them, thump, thump, thump. And he came, he came, he came, he really came—he shot everything right up my ass, and I had another orgasm, and then we hugged tight together and we hugged and we hugged and neither of us wanted to let go, never."

When he was using a camcorder, Jeff was able to focus on what it was about June that excited him, and to see that she was just as exciting as a commercial sex video—more so, because he knew her, she was real, and he could actually make love to her once the video was over. He had been afraid of a real-life sexual encounter (after all, once you've closed a porno magazine, the sexual experience is over, and you don't have to worry about the continuing welfare of the girls who have excited you so much). But making his first sex video had shown him that he had the best of all possible worlds.

June said, "We've made a whole lot more videos since, and sometimes we lie in bed and watch them and make love. To be honest, I think the really dirty ones are the most exciting. Jeff took one of me masturbating with this huge carrot we found at the market . . . and then there's another sequence with Jeff masturbating in the living room, lying on his back, so that when he comes, the sperm shoots all over him, all over his stomach. He wipes it all off with his hand and then he licks it. That really turned me on, Jeff swallowing his own sperm.

"Making sexy videos has helped us to break down all of our sexual inhibitions, do you know what I mean? These days, we're not shy about anything. We do it as a game, kind of a contest between us, who can make the sexiest video. You ought to tell people to try it, it's very, very sexy and it's fantastic fun. The dirtiest one is one we filmed in the yard together. We set the camcorder up on a clamp—you don't have to buy a whole tripod, you can just buy a clamp which you can attach to a chairback or anything.

"I'm lying naked on the sunbed, massaging myself with sun oil. I smear it all over my breasts and stomach, and then massage it between my legs. Then Jeff appears and he's naked, too, and his cock's already hard. He stands next to me, and I take hold of his cock in my hand and rub it for him, then I take it into my mouth and start to suck it. You can even see it making the side of my cheek bulge!

"Jeff climbs onto the sunbed and I open up my legs for him, and he slides his cock into my pussy. He fucks me very, very slowly, and just before he climaxes, he takes his cock out of me and shoots three big squirts of sperm all over my pussy, and then he rubs it in with his fingers.

"I keep on massaging his sperm into my pussy, while he stands up again, and stands next to me. The sound isn't very good, but you can just hear him saying, 'Shall I piss on you?' and I take hold of his cock in my hand and kiss it and suck the last of the sperm off it. Then he starts to piss, over my breasts at first. That was the first time I had ever done anything like that, and it turned me on so much I felt breathless. You can see me in the video, frantically masturbating myself, while

Jeff is pissing all over my breasts, first one nipple, then the other, and the piss is pouring off my nipples and down my stomach. Then I take hold of his cock in my hand, and aim it right at my face. I'll never forget what that felt like, the first time, all that hot clear piss splashing all over my face. I opened my mouth so that he could piss straight into it, and I swallowed and swallowed. It tasted kind of salty-sweet, but delicious, too. It's addictive, if you ask me! When he'd finished pissing, I still couldn't get enough of the taste, and you can see me sucking at his cock and his balls as if I'm going to swallow them. Jeff starts to get another hard-on.

"I open my legs and he kneels down between them and starts to kiss and lick my pussy, and slide his fingers up it. That's when I decide to get my own back! I reach down and pull the lips of my pussy apart. At first nothing happens—I was so excited I couldn't get myself started! Then I start to piss, too, a thin high jet of piss—you don't even realize how far a woman can do it until you see it done like that. You can see Jeff turning his face from one side to the other, so that I'm pissing all over his face, and the piss dripping from his eyelashes and his chin. Then he opens his mouth and presses it right over my pussy. You can see his adam's apple working up and down as he swallows. When I've finished, he climbs on top of me, and his cock's enormous, and he fucks me again. That's my favorite video, for sure.

"Do I think it's disgusting? Of course not. Jeff and I are both clean, healthy people. What we do together to show our love for each other is our own business. We enjoy it. We love it! And I can tell you something— if more women were willing to be a little bit naughtier, like me, than fewer women would lose their men.

"You don't serve up the same dinner, night after night. You don't wear the same clothes, day after day.

Think how boring that would be! It's the same with sex. Why not try something new? I know it can be kind of embarrassing when you do something different for the first time, but the fun it gives you, and the love it brings you . . . well, there's no describing how good it is."

Sue-Ann, 27, a catering assistant from Tampa, Florida, produced a home video with her new husband, Paul, 31, which served not only as an erotic stimulus for lovemaking, but as a romantic reminder of their wedding.

"We decided to make a 'wedding-night' video. It's very sexy, but it's very beautiful and emotional, too. The day after the wedding, our whole apartment was filled with flowers, so it makes a fantastic background. The video starts with me coming into the living-room in my bridal gown, complete with veil and a bouquet of pink-and-white flowers. It was a fabulous gown, all white silk with tiny seed pearls sewn on the bodice. I look so virginal!

"Then Paul comes into the room, dressed in his morning suit and wing collar and everything, and lifts up my veil and kisses me. That's definitely one of my favorite scenes. Next, we go into the bedroom. Paul kisses me again, and then he takes off all of his clothes. He looks terrific—he has a very athletic body, and his cock is sticking out, and that turns me on so much, that scene!

"He kisses me and caresses my breasts through my silk bodice. Then he lifts up my gown and my petticoats, and you can see for the first time that I'm wearing white stockings, held up with a white garter-belt, and no panties. I keep my gown and my petticoats lifted up, and Paul kneels down between my legs and starts to kiss and lick my pussy. We did a close-up of that, and even though it's very erotic, it's very beautiful, too. Paul is surrounded by all this white frothy net and silk, with his tongue licking my bright pink pussy.

"Then he lifts me up, like he's carrying me over the threshold, and lays me down on the bed, with my gown still raised. He kneels on the pillow next to me, and I take hold of his cock and kiss it and suck it and curl my tongue all around it. Then he lifts up his cock with his hand and I take his balls into my mouth, one after the other, and lick deep between his legs.

"After that, he opens up my legs. It's such a fantastic scene . . . I'm wearing this gorgeous white bridal gown, complete with stockings and white satin slippers, and yet you can see absolutely *everything*! But of course wedding nights are like that—romantic, but very, very sexy, too! At last you're allowed to do it legally!

"You can see me lying back on the bed, surrounded by lilies and roses and carnations, still wearing my veil. I'm holding my pussy wide open with both hands, and Paul kneels down in between my knees and fits the head of his cock into it, and then slides it in so slowly it looks like slow motion.

"We make love really luxuriously. You can see Paul's cock sliding in and out of me, all glistening and red. You can see my face, too, and it looks like I'm having the time of my life! Then Paul comes, and he takes out his cock so that his come drops onto my pussy. You see these white drops, and my white stockings, and my white bridal gown, and it's truly fantastic."

Finally—let's take a look at one of the most important ways in which you can make yourself sexually irresistible to the man you love—and that's to use *spontaneous compliments and displays of affection*: It has often surprised me how many couples fall out of the habit of flirting with each other. Just because they've been married for a few years, each of them seems to assume that their sexual interest in the other is "understood," and doesn't need constant re-expression. How many times have you heard a hurt-sounding husband protesting "But you *know* I love you. Of *course* I think you're sexy! I wouldn't still be here if I didn't!"

And how many times have you heard a woman refer to her husband's sexual ability in mildly scornful terms, not because she *really* thinks that he's not much good in bed, but because she's embarrassed to say that he's a wonderful lover. Yet what do you think he would really prefer to hear?

If you've enjoyed your lovemaking, pay your lover a compliment by telling him how good it was. Tell him how he makes you feel. Try to describe what your orgasm was like, if you had one. Ask him how his climax felt. Compliment him on the size of his penis, and the amount of sperm he ejaculated. "You must have shot out so much . . . I could actually feel it inside me."

First and last rule of making a man feel sexually good about himself: *You can never, ever flatter him too much about his sexual prowess.* The man isn't born who doesn't warm to compliments about his skills in bed and his physical attractiveness.

Don't leave the sexual flattery behind in the bedroom. It never hurts to make a point of looking dreamy during the day, and, when you're asked what you're thinking about, to say something like "The way you made love to me last night."

Another erotic compliment is to whisper to him, when you come out of the ladies' restroom, "I just went to the bathroom . . . and I could still smell you . . . and there's no smell like it in the world."

Intimate touching is another way of reminding him that he turns you on. Come up behind him when he's cooking or washing the car and give him a provocative squeeze through his pants. Do it when you're watching television together in the evening, or even, if you feel like it, open up his zipper, take out his cock and give him a few moments of teasing oral sex. He won't forget it and you won't regret it.

Ellie, 34, a grade-school teacher from New York City, told me: "My first marriage died of neglect. He neglected me and I neglected him. When we divorced, I suddenly realized that I *had* loved him all those years, but I'd never told him. I'd never said, 'I think you're so good looking,' or, 'I think you're terrific in bed,' even though he was. Of course he never paid me compliments, either, but two wrongs don't make a right, and if I'd made a habit of complimenting *him*, then maybe he would have made a habit of complimenting *me*.

"By the time I realized what had gone wrong with our marriage, it was too late. David had found another woman. But I promised myself that I would never let it happen again. I went through three years of loneliness before I met Ted, and now that I've found him I'm going to keep him! I'm always paying him compliments, I'm always touching him. I'm always showing him that I love him and that he turns me on."

Your caresses don't necessarily have to be blatantly sexual. Stroking your lover's hair while he's sitting beside you reading a book is enough to show how much you care for him. Squeezing his knee when he's driving. Kissing him on the top of the head while he's eating his breakfast.

You can encourage him to touch you, too, and that will keep his level of sexual interest high. Take hold of his hand and press it against your breast. Do the housework wearing nothing but one of his shirts, and see if he can resist touching you between the legs.

Think of little sexy things you can do for him. When he comes home from work, wear a deeply unbuttoned blouse with no bra underneath. When he leaves for work the next morning, slip one of your G-strings into his pants pocket—one of your *used* G-strings. Call him at work and tell him that you're thinking about his cock and that you can't wait for him to get home.

Make it a habit to be complimentary and sexy all the time, and you will reap the benefits in a long and passionate relationship. Everything else being equal, you will continue to be sexy, you will continue to be wild . . . but you won't ever have to be single, ever again.

TEN

Want a New Lover? Twenty-Five Things You Can Do Right Now

1. Look at yourself in the mirror. Tell yourself the truth: that you're sexy and that you're special and that any man would be proud to call you his lover.

2. Write down a description of yourself—who you are, what you are, how old you are, your height, weight, hair color, eye color, ethnic grouping. Describe your education, your career, your marital status.

3. Write down your greatest *immediate* ambition, apart from finding a new sex partner. Lose weight? Make money? Have your hair fixed? Take a weekend vacation? Have dinner at a gourmet restaurant? Anything that you think would make you feel better.

4. Whatever you wrote for (3), arrange to do it within the next 24 hours. No matter what it is, *do* it.

5. Write down the real reason you don't have a current sex partner. Be totally honest with yourself.

6. Write down the kind of man you would ideally like as a sex partner. Be selective. Be *very* selective. Age? Looks? Profession? Marital status? Income? Smoking or nonsmoking? Sporty or

slothful? Intellectual or regular-strength brain? Children? Animals? Ambitions? Don't compromise on your ideals. When you eventually find a man you really like, you'll find that he doesn't match up to every criterion in any case.

7. Is there a man you already know whom you would like as a sexual partner? If so, make up your mind that you're not going to be frightened; you're going to call him or meet him and tell him how you feel.

8. Ask yourself whether you're looking for a series of short but exciting sexual experiences, or a long-term, stable sexual relationship.

9. Ask yourself if you would be prepared to change your life totally in order to find a long-term sex partner. Would you relocate, and if so, how far? Would you change jobs? Give up your job altogether? Take on stepchildren?

10. Decide on your plan of action: Are you going to look for a man in the personal columns? Are you going to place a personal ad yourself? Are you going to join a personal introduction agency? What about a lunch club? Make up your mind what you're going to do, and *do* it. Today.

11. Make a comprehensive assessment of yourself. Do you like your hair/makeup/nails? If not, arrange to have them fixed so that you're completely happy with them. *Don't worry about your weight*. In all of my years of sex counseling, I have always strongly advised women against dieting while they're trying to find a new lover or to establish a new sexual relationship. Just don't bother. You'll be much more emotionally relaxed. You'll be yourself. Men are much less worried about a woman's weight than women think they are. In fact, 63 percent of men I surveyed two years ago said that they preferred

plumper women. Another 11 percent said that they were really turned on by fat women. So forget dieting. Eat normally and healthily, and you'll find that your weight remains pretty stable, anyway.

12. Plan a new wardrobe. Make a list of all the clothes you need to make up a smart and interesting new wardrobe. Work out which clothes are really essential, and make sure that you buy them within 48 hours, even if you can't afford everything you need.

13. Think what erotic underwear you'd like to buy. Be bold and sexy and indulge yourself. Make a list and send off for a catalog.

14. Give yourself all of those cosmetic treatments you've been putting off for so long. Give yourself a face-pack, wax your legs, shave your armpits, trim or shave off your pubic hair. Make yourself immaculate.

15. Do you think your conversation is limited? At the very least, read a copy of *Time* or *Newsweek* and *Readers Digest*. Follow up on some of the topics these magazines raise. Read some of the books they review. Make up your mind to go see some of the plays or concerts or movies. Try to remember one or two of the true stories or jokes out of *Readers Digest*. They may not be particularly brilliant, but it's good practice, trying to remember anecdotes for use in conversation. Suddenly you'll find that you've always got something amusing to say, and you can say goodbye to those awkward silences.

16. Learn about sex and lovemaking. Read this book over and try to read more, such as *How to Drive Your Man Wild in Bed* and *More Ways to Drive Your Man Wild in Bed*.

17. Write down (in note form, if you like) your fa-

vorite sexual fantasy. Making love to Richard Gere and Tom Cruise, both at the same time? Being a dominatrix and whipping defenseless men? Starring in a strip show?

18. Make a list of any sexual variations that you've never tried before, and which you'd really like to try (with the right man, of course). Oral sex? Anal sex? Mutual masturbation? Bondage? Sex outdoors?

19. Make a list of any sexual variation that you would *never* want to do. Ask yourself *why* you would never want to do it and how you would react if a man you really liked asked you to do it.

20. Make a list of all the sex toys you would be interested in trying, and send off for a mail-order catalog so that you can try them. Be brave. It's your sex life, nobody else's.

21. Learn as much as you can about your body and your sexual responses. Look at your vulva in the mirror. Identify your clitoris, your urethra, your vagina, your inner lips. Masturbate in the mirror and watch how your vulva changes color, how your lubricating juices start to flow, and how your lips begin to swell.

22. Draw up a chart of sexual self-stimulation. Masturbate today, and at least once every day, and note down how long it took you to reach orgasm. Make a note, too, of how you stimulated yourself. (Did you use your fingers alone, or a dildo, or other object? Did you use a magazine or a video to give you extra excitement?) Did you have an erotic fantasy while you masturbated? If so, what was it?

23. Make up your mind that this is the day that is going to change your life. Finding an exciting new lover is not an impossible dream. It's something that you can start doing now. There are

dozens of agencies and clubs and dating services that can help you to find the right person, as long as *you* have the courage to try them.

24. Decide that you're not going to allow embarrassment or inhibition or lack of knowledge to affect your sex life ever again. You're going to be sexy, wild, and happy, too.

25. Promise that you'll write and tell me when you've found the lover you've always wanted.

And, Last of All, Single Women and AIDS

One of the most inhibiting factors when you're looking for a new lover is the fear that he may be HIV-positive—in other words, that he may be carrying the virus that causes AIDS.

The single most effective protection against the transmission of AIDS is the condom, or sheath, and if you decide to have intercourse with a man whose sexual history you're not 100 percent sure of, then you must insist that he wear one. I'm not talking about "suggest" or "ask" or "recommend." I'm talking about *"insist."*

These days, you should never feel embarrassed about insisting that your lover wear a condom. You're not implying that he is actually HIV-positive. You're simply taking a sensible precaution. Besides that, condoms protect against the transmission of all venereal diseases, including gonorrhea, herpes and non-specific urethritis (NSU).

Equally important, they protect against unwanted pregnancy.

If your would-be lover refuses to wear a condom, then you will have to say "no"—no matter how much he argues and no matter how much you want to make love to him. Your life is worth more than his momentary pleasure.

If your lover really hates condoms, then you do have an alternative in the Femidom, or female condom. The female condom is a disposable sheath that you insert like a tampon before making love and remove afterward whenever you choose. It is made out of polyurethane, rather than latex rubber, so it doesn't smell like most male condoms.

The female condom has an inner ring that helps you to insert it, and an outer ring that is pushed flat against your vaginal lips to prevent it from being drawn inside the vagina during lovemaking. Compared to male condoms, it's quite soft and comfortable, and you can lubricate it with body juices or KY jelly or Vaseline (unlike male condoms, which should never be lubricated with oil-based products.)

After lovemaking, you twist the outer ring of the male condom to prevent sperm from escaping, draw it out of your vagina, and dispose of it. The only complaints I have heard about it is that it tends to move during intercourse.

HIV is found in the bloodstream, and in the fluids that are exchanged during sexual intercourse (men's pre-ejaculatory juice and semen, and women's lubricating juices). There is no record of it ever having been passed on by kissing, even deep French kissing.

You can protect yourself and prevent the spread of AIDS if you *always* use a condom when you have sex with somebody whose sexual history is questionable. You should take particular care when having anal intercourse, since the rectal tissues sometimes tear slightly and infected semen could pass the virus directly and immediately into your bloodstream. If you are considering anal sex with a new lover, you should make sure that you buy extra-strong condoms.

The virus can also be passed on to either partner by

unprotected vaginal intercourse. Always wear a condom. If you don't have a condom, don't do it.

There is a theoretical risk of catching the virus through oral sex, particularly if you have open cuts or ulcers in your mouth. There is also a risk from sharing sex toys like vibrators.

On the whole, though, the etiquette of AIDS is simply this: You are entitled to expect your new lover to wear a condom, and he, in turn, should never make an issue of it. If he likes you enough to want to make love to you, then he should also like you enough to protect you from the risk of disease and pregnancy.

The most sophisticated and sensible answer is always to have a large dish of assorted condoms beside the bed, rather like a dish of jellybeans. Just like jellybeans, condoms will make life even sweeter.

Before you agree to a live-in sexual relationship, you are perfectly entitled to ask your lover to take an AIDS test. I know this won't be the easiest of precautions to suggest to him, but you can take some of the sting out of it by agreeing to take a simultaneous test yourself. Tell him that you love him, that both of your lives are too valuable to risk, and that you want to be 100 percent confident and relaxed when you make love together.

An AIDS test is essential if your new relationship is beginning to look serious and you've started thinking about children. Because it is carried in the bloodstream, the AIDS virus is *always* passed on by HIV-positive mothers to their babies in the womb.

While this may end a book of erotic pleasure on a serious note, new research indicates that the incidence of HIV among heterosexuals is leveling out, and in some countries is even beginning to show signs of decline. This is a direct result of safe and sensible sex practices, and of women insisting that even if they're single, sexy and wild, they still want to be safe.

Good luck, good-looking, and good loving.

There's an epidemic with 27 million victims. And no visible symptoms.

It's an epidemic of people who can't read.

Believe it or not, 27 million Americans are functionally illiterate, about one adult in five.

The solution to this problem is you... when you join the fight against illiteracy. So call the Coalition for Literacy at toll-free **1-800-228-8813** and volunteer.

Volunteer Against Illiteracy. The only degree you need is a degree of caring.